Leg Pain in the Running Athlete

Guest Editor

ALEXANDER K. MEININGER, MD

CLINICS IN SPORTS MEDICINE

www.sportsmed.theclinics.com

Consulting Editor
MARK D. MILLER, MD

April 2012 • Volume 31 • Number 2

SAUNDERS an imprint of ELSEVIER, Inc.

W.B. SAUNDERS COMPANY
A Division of Elsevier Inc.

1600 John F. Kennedy Blvd. • Suite 1800 • Philadelphia, Pennsylvania 19103

http://www.theclinics.com

CLINICS IN SPORTS MEDICINE Volume 31, Number 2
April 2012 ISSN 0278-5919, ISBN-13: 978-1-4557-3936-3

Editor: Jessica McCool
Developmental Editor: Teia Stone

Photocopying

Single photocopies of single articles may be made for personal use as allowed by national copyright laws. Permission of the Publisher and payment of a fee is required for all other photocopying, including multiple or systematic copying, copying for advertising or promotional purposes, resale, and all forms of document delivery. Special rates are available for educational institutions that wish to make photocopies for non-profit educational classroom use. For information on how to seek permission visit www.elsevier.com/permissions or call: (+44) 1865 843830 (UK)/(+1) 215 239 3804 (USA).

Derivative Works

Subscribers may reproduce tables of contents or prepare lists of articles including abstracts for internal circulation within their institutions. Permission of the Publisher is required for resale or distribution outside the institution. Permission of the Publisher is required for all other derivative works, including compilations and translations (please consult www.elsevier.com/permissions).

Electronic Storage or Usage

Permission of the Publisher is required to store or use electronically any material contained in this journal, including any article or part of an article (please consult www.elsevier.com/permissions). Except as outlined above, no part of this publication may be reproduced, stored in a retrieval system or transmitted in any form or by any means, electronic, mechanical, photocopying, recording or otherwise, without prior written permission of the Publisher.

Notice

No responsibility is assumed by the Publisher for any injury and/or damage to persons or property as a matter of products liability, negligence or otherwise, or from any use or operation of any methods, products, instructions or ideas contained in the material herein. Because of rapid advances in the medical sciences, in particular, independent verification of diagnoses and drug dosages should be made.

Although all advertising material is expected to conform to ethical (medical) standards, inclusion in this publication does not constitute a guarantee or endorsement of the quality or value of such product or of the claims made of it by its manufacturer.

Clinics in Sports Medicine (ISSN 0278-5919) is published quarterly by Elsevier Inc., 360 Park Avenue South, New York, NY 10010-1710. Months of issue are January, April, July, and October. Business and Editorial Offices: 1600 John F. Kennedy Blvd., Ste. 1800, Philadelphia, PA 19103-2899. Customer Service Office: 3251 Riverport Lane, Maryland Heights, MO 63043. Periodicals postage paid at New York, NY and additional mailing offices. Subscription prices are $324.00 per year (US individuals), $503.00 per year (US institutions), $160.00 per year (US students), $367.00 per year (Canadian individuals), $608.00 per year (Canadian institutions), $223.00 (Canadian students), $446.00 per year (foreign individuals), $608.00 per year (foreign institutions), and $223.00 per year (foreign students). Foreign air speed delivery is included in all *Clinics* subscription prices. All prices are subject to change without notice. **POSTMASTER:** Send address changes to *Clinics in Sports Medicine,* Elsevier Health Sciences Division, Subscription Customer Service, 3251 Riverport Lane, Maryland Heights, MO 63043. Customer Service (orders, claims, online, change of address): Elsevier Health Sciences Division, Subscription Customer Service, 3251 Riverport Lane, Maryland Heights, MO 63043. Tel: 1-800-654-2452 (U.S. and Canada); 314-447-8871 (outside U.S. and Canada). Fax: 314-447-8029. E-mail: journalscustomerservice-usa@elsevier.com (for print support); journalsonlinesupport-usa@elsevier.com (for online support).

Reprints. For copies of 100 or more of articles in this publication, please contact the Commercial Reprints Department, Elsevier Inc., 360 Park Avenue South, New York, NY 10010-1710. Tel.: 212-633-3812; Fax: 212-462-1935; E-mail: reprints@elsevier.com.

Clinics in Sports Medicine is covered in *MEDLINE/PubMed (Index Medicus) Current Contents/Clinical Medicine, Excerpta Medica,* and *ISI/Biomed.*

Printed and bound by CPI Group (UK) Ltd, Croydon, CR0 4YY

Transferred to Digital Print 2012

Contributors

CONSULTING EDITOR

MARK D. MILLER, MD
S. Ward Casscells Professor of Orthopaedic Surgery, University of Virginia, Charlottesville, Virginia; Team Physician, James Madison University, Harrisonburg, Virginia

GUEST EDITOR

ALEXANDER K. MEININGER, MD
Orthopaedic Surgery and Sports Medicine, Moab Regional Specialty Clinic, Moab, Utah

AUTHORS

KASHIF ALI, MD
Orthopaedic Surgery Resident, University of Chicago, Chicago, Illinois

MICHAEL BRESLER, MD
Assistant Clinical Professor of Radiology, University of Illinois at Chicago Medical Center, Chicago, Illinois

CHARLES A. BUSH-JOSEPH, MD
Professor, Department of Orthopedic Surgery, Rush University Medical Center, Chicago, Illinois

JAY F. DEIMEL, MD
Orthopaedic Surgery Resident, Section of Orthopaedic Surgery, and Rehabilitation Medicine, University of Chicago Medical Center, Chicago, Illinois

BRADLEY J. DUNLAP, MD
Orthopaedic Surgeon, NorthShore University HealthSystem, Evanston; Clinical Instructor, University of Chicago Pritzker School of Medicine, Chicago, Illinois

AMIR EL SHAMI, MD
Sports Medicine Fellow, Physical Medicine and Rehabilitation, Family Medicine Department, University of Illinois at Chicago, Chicago, Illinois

CHRISTOPHER A. GEORGE, MD
Resident Physician, Department of Orthopaedic Surgery, University of Illinois Hospital at Chicago, Chicago, Illinois

DAVID R. GUELICH, MD, COSM
Assistant Professor of Orthopedic Surgery, Department of Orthopedics, University of Illinois Medical Center, University of Illinois at Chicago Medical School, Chicago, Illinois

SHERWIN S.W. HO, MD
Director, Sports Medicine Fellowship, Associate Professor, Department of Surgery, Section of Orthopaedics and Rehabilitation, University of Chicago Hospital, Chicago, Illinois

MARK R. HUTCHINSON, MD
Professor, Director of Sports Medicine, Department of Orthopaedic Surgery, University of Illinois Hospital at Chicago, Chicago, Illinois

DAVID J. JEWISON, MD
MacNeal Sports Medicine Fellowship, Chicago, Illinois

JASON L. KOH, MD
Vice Chairman, Department of Orthopaedic Surgery, NorthShore University HealthSystem, Evanston, Illinois

J. MARTIN LELAND, MD
Orthopaedic Sports Medicine; Assistant Professor, Department of Orthopaedic Surgery, University of Chicago, Chicago, Illinois

PAUL B. LEWIS, MD, MS
Department of Diagnostic Radiology and Nuclear Medicine, Rush University Medical Center, Chicago, Illinois

WINNIE MAR, MD
Assistant Clinical Professor of Radiology, University of Illinois at Chicago Medical Center, Chicago, Illinois

LCDR FRANK MCCORMICK, MD, MC, USNR
Resident in Orthopaedic Surgery, Harvard Combined Orthopedic Residency Program, Boston, Massachusetts

ALEXANDER K. MEININGER, MD
Orthopaedic Surgery and Sports Medicine, Moab Regional Specialty Clinic, Moab, Utah

TERRY L. NICOLA, MD, MS
Fellowship Director, Sports Medicine; Director, Sports Medicine Rehabilitation; Assistant Professor, Clinical Rehabilitation Medicine, Department of Orthopedic Surgery; Adjunct Professor, Family Medicine Department, University of Illinois at Chicago, Chicago, Illinois

BENEDICT U. NWACHUKWU, BA
Medical Student, Harvard Medical School, Boston, Massachusetts

CDR MATTHEW T. PROVENCHER, MD, MC, USN
Attending Orthopaedic Surgeon, Director of Orthopaedic Shoulder and Sports Surgery, Naval Medical Center San Diego, San Diego, California

NOAM RESHEF, MD
Fellow, Orthopedic Sports Medicine, Center for Athletic Medicine and the University of Illinois at Chicago, Chicago, Illinois

DEANA RUBY, APN, ACNP-BC
Advanced Practice Nurse, Department of Orthopedic Surgery, Rush University Medical Center, Chicago, Illinois

CHRISTIAN C. SKJONG, MD
Resident Physician, Department of Surgery, Section of Orthopaedics and Rehabilitation, University of Chicago Hospital, Chicago, Illinois

JORDAN TOMAN, MD
Department of Radiology, University of Illinois at Chicago Medical Center, Chicago, Illinois

WILLIAM D. TURNIPSEED, MD
Professor of Surgery, Division of Vascular Surgery, Department of Surgery, University of Wisconsin School of Medicine and Public Health, Madison, Wisconsin

Contents

The Anatomy and Biomechanics of Running   187

Terry L. Nicola and David J. Jewison

> The series of kinematic and kinetic events during the running movement is reviewed. The focus is more on the kinetic chain of the lower extremities during stance phase and swing phase of running. A literature review will use this knowledge base of kinematic and kinetic events to compare variations in anatomy, which have been identified as risk factors for injury. Pelvis, torso, and upper extremity contributions to the running movement are included in this review.

Evaluation of the Injured Runner   203

Alexander K. Meininger and Jason L. Koh

> Running is a complex biomechanical task that places unique strain on the musculoskeletal system. Injuries in runners are most commonly related to overuse or abrupt changes in training habits. Risk factors for injury include biomechanical malalignment or strength deficiencies. Weakness at any point in the kinetic chain places athletes at risk. The evaluation depends on a thorough history, comprehensive physical examination, and functional testing to recognize and prevent injury.

Diagnostic Imaging in the Evaluation of Leg Pain in Athletes   217

Michael Bresler, Winnie Mar, and Jordan Toman

> Diagnostic imaging is an important tool in the evaluation of athletes with both chronic and acute leg pain. Radiologic evaluation can confirm injury, aid in clinical management decisions, and help determine prognosis and time required before return to sport. The radiologic appearance and imaging modalities of choice for evaluating stress injuries to bone, hamstring, and Achilles injuries; chronic exertional compartment syndrome; and popliteal artery entrapment syndrome are reviewed.

> The Female Athlete Triad is a syndrome of 3 interrelated conditions including energy deficit, menstrual dysfunction, and altered bone mineral density. With the increasing number of female athletes since the passage of Title IX, the triad continues to alter the well being of this enlarging population. A number of female athletes, including distance runners, are at heightened risk for this condition. This article serves to define the spectrum of components within the triad as well as review methodology for proper evaluation, treatment, and prevention of this syndrome.

> Immediate and delayed-onset muscle soreness differ mainly in chronology of presentation. Both conditions share the same quality of pain, provoking and relieving activities as well as the variable degree of functional deficits. There is no single mechanism for muscle soreness; instead, it is a culmination of six different mechanisms. The several modalities to manage the associated symptoms of muscle soreness have outcomes that seem to be as diverse as the modalities themselves. The clinical presentation, cellular mechanism and selected treatment modalities are reviewed in this communication.

> Hamstring injuries are quite common among the modern day athlete. The high recurrence rate and, at times, prolonged recovery associated with these injuries make them particularly challenging. Most low-grade strains are treated conservatively, whereas patients with complete ruptures off the ischium may benefit from surgical management, given the appropriate clinical setting. This article discusses the diagnosis and treatment of hamstring injuries as well as a review of the current literature and a suggested rehabilitation protocol following proximal hamstring repairs.

> Medial tibial stress syndrome (MTSS) is a common problem among runners, military recruits, and dancers, although it may affect any type of endurance athlete. MTSS is commonly thought to be an overuse problem and was thought to be the first stage of stress fracture. Basic science studies reveal a combination of forces acting along an area of poor vascularity and tissue compliance. Diagnosis is clinical, and imaging studies may assist in ruling out other causes of pain. Treatment

options are numerous; however, studies have not shown major advantage to any specific treatment regiment.

A cumulative trauma model is used to review the nonsurgical treatment of running injuries. This includes acute and recurrent injuries, with associated chronic changes to muscle, ligament, tendon, and bone. General concepts are reviewed for initial protection, relative rest, and treatment of inflammation. These concepts are then combined with strategies used for the rehabilitation of specific injuries in a patient population very reluctant to take any time off from running and exercise.

VISIT THE CLINICS ONLINE!

Access your subscription at:
www.theclinics.com

Foreword

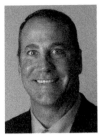

Mark D. Miller, MD
Consulting Editor

One could argue that the limping athlete is more difficult to diagnose and treat than the limping child. There are a variety of conditions that can cause leg pain in the athlete and these often coexist and represent a significant challenge. As we all know, runners want only one thing—to return to running. Unfortunately, many of these conditions require prolonged treatment and rehabilitation, so that goal is often not immediately achieved. Dr Alexander Meininger from the Moab Regional Specialty Clinic in Moab, Utah has put together an excellent treatise on leg pain in running athletes. This edition has a very organized format, beginning with anatomy and proceeding to evaluation and then treatment of each condition. The issue concludes with an excellent review of rehabilitation. The running athlete is a major challenge to us all, but hopefully this issue will provide some insight that will make our job just a little easier.

Mark D. Miller, MD
S. Ward Casscells Professor of Orthopaedic Surgery
University of Virginia
Team Physician, James Madison University
400 Ray C. Hunt Drive, Suite 330
Charlottesville, VA 22908-0159, USA

E-mail address:
mdm3p@virginia.edu

Clin Sports Med 31 (2012) xi
doi:10.1016/j.csm.2012.01.001
0278-5919/12/$ – see front matter

Preface

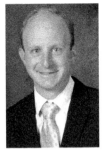

Alexander K. Meininger, MD
Guest Editor

Leg pain in the running athlete can be a complicated and frustrating experience for the athlete and physician alike. Myriad of clinical conditions is complicated by the diverse and disparate diagnoses captured under the wastebasket term "shin splints." This issue is designed to provide the sports medicine clinician or surgeon our most current understanding of the pathophysiology behind leg pain in runners.

The first article is written by one of our foremost leaders in running medicine, researcher, and Sports Medicine Rehabilitation director Dr Terry Nicola. He eloquently summarizes the biomechanics of running as a basis for understanding pathology. I am thrilled to engage my mentor Dr Jason Koh in the next article, who describes our routine for evaluating running injuries clinically, while Dr Bresler and his team write a wonderful summary of the radiologic findings unique to leg pain.

Subsequent articles breaking down the differential diagnoses discuss muscle cramps, hamstring injuries, medial tibial stress syndrome, exertional compartment syndrome, and popliteal artery entrapment by Drs Bush-Joseph, Leland, Guelich, Hutchinson, and Turnipseed. Tendinopathy treatment is a hot topic in sports medicine today and I am honored to have Dr Sherwin Ho's expertise to examine the evidence for treatment. Obviously no discussion of leg pain would be complete without recognizing stress fractures and the role of the female athlete triad and I am indebted to Drs Provencher and Dunlap for their insights.

None of this would have been possible without the dedication, time, and effort of my contributing authors. I want to give special thanks to Dr Mark Miller for granting me the opportunity to participate in the *Clinics in Sports Medicine*, as well as Jessica McCool from Elsevier for keeping us on schedule. Last, to my beautiful wife, Angie—I couldn't have done it without your support and understanding, thank you.

Clin Sports Med 31 (2012) xiii–xiv
doi:10.1016/j.csm.2012.01.002
0278-5919/12/$ – see front matter © 2012 Elsevier Inc. All rights reserved.

sportsmed.theclinics.com

It is my pleasure to share this work with you. I hope that you'll enjoy reading this issue as much as I enjoyed assembling it.

Alexander K. Meininger, MD
Orthopaedic Surgery and Sports Medicine
Moab Regional Specialty Clinic
476 West Williams Way, Suite B
Moab, UT 84532, USA

E-mail address:
DrAlex@mrhmoab.org

The Anatomy and Biomechanics of Running

Terry L. Nicola, MD, MS[a,b,c],*, David J. Jewison, MD[d]

KEYWORDS

• Running • Biomechanics • Gait cycle • Running injuries

The study of the biomechanics of running refers to understanding the structure, function, and capability of the lower extremities and overall kinetic chain that allow a human to run. Although no two individuals share identical anatomy, strength, or proprioceptive qualities, there are many similarities to understand regarding the role of each individual's running cycle to diagnose and treat injuries that occur from running. This article discusses the anatomy of the lower extremity as it relates to the ability to run, the running gait cycle, and abnormal anatomy and biomechanics related to running injuries.

RUNNING GAIT CYCLE

The running gait cycle is different from the walking gait cycle. The gait cycle can be described as the series of movements of the lower extremities between foot initial impact with the surface until it reconnects with the surface at the end of the cycle.[1] To better understand the gait cycle, we examine the walking gait cycle and its differences from the running gait cycle. There are 2 main phases of the gait cycle, the stance phase and the swing phase.[1–3,4] The stance phase occurs during the period of contact between the foot and the running or walking surface. These phases occur in both walking and running. When one lower extremity is in the stance phase, the other is in the swing phase (**Figs. 1–3**).

Running is distinct from walking because of an additional float phase, which occurs twice during running. This float phase occurs between stance phase and the swing phase, where both lower extremities are not in contact with the ground.[1] Therefore, running at any speed can be defined as either 1 leg or no leg striking the ground throughout the gait cycle. During the walking cycle, there is a period of double stance

The authors have nothing to disclose.
a UIC Sports Medicine Center, 839 West Roosevelt Avenue, Suite #102, Chicago, IL 60608, USA
b Department of Orthopedic Surgery, University of Illinois at Chicago, Chicago, IL, USA
c Family Medicine Department, University of Illinois at Chicago, Chicago, IL, USA
d MacNeal Sports Medicine, 125 East 13th Street 615, Chicago, IL 60605, USA
* Corresponding author. UIC Sports Medicine Center, 839 West Roosevelt Avenue, Suite #102, Chicago, IL 60608.
E-mail address: tnicola@uic.edu

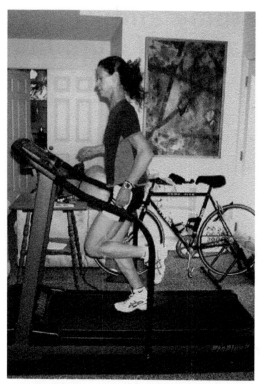

Fig. 1. Swing and stance phases of running. Right leg in stance phase, left leg in swing phase.

phase during the walking gait cycle in which both lower extremities are in contact with the walking surface.[2] This occurs for walking at the very beginning and very end of the stance phase. This means that during walking, 1 or 2 legs are always in contact with the ground during stance phase.[1] For walking, stance phase occurs typically for about 60% of the gait cycle, and swing phase occurs for about 40% of the cycle.[1,2] For walking, stance phase occurs in greater than 50% of the cycle, with swing phase consisting of the rest of the cycle.[3] The opposite is true for running, in which stance phase is less than 50% of the cycle.[2,5] This swing phase for greater than 50% of the cycle causes an overlap of swing phases between lower extremities, generating the characteristic float phase. As velocity in running increases, stance phase becomes even less of a percentage of the cycle.[2] Therefore, sprinters spend a smaller percentage of the gait cycle in stance phase. Additionally, step length and cadence are increased during running compared to walking.[2,5] Stride length is the distance from initial contact of 1 foot until the same foot makes contact with the running surface again. Step length is the distance between initial contact of one foot and the subsequent initial contact of the opposite foot. Cadence is the number of steps taken during a certain amount of time. As running cadence, stride, and step length increase, velocity and ground reaction forces increase.[2,5] This has implications for increased stresses through the lower extremities and risk for injury. One other difference is that walking has a wider base between individual footstrikes. This is the distance between medial borders of the heels. Walking has a greater base width of support, approximately 1 inch, than running. As speed increases into a run, the base of support

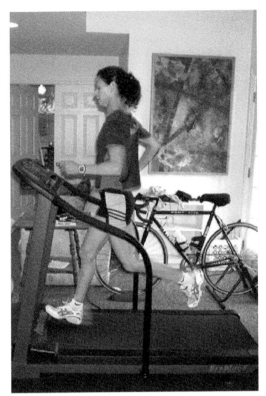

Fig. 2. Swing and stance phases of running. Right leg footstrike, end of float phase, beginning of swing phase left leg.

narrows so that foot strike is more on the centerline of progression. Hip rotation in the transverse plane reduces the up and down fall of the center of gravity.[2,4] Additional differences between walking and running worth mentioning here are that running requires a greater range of motion of all lower limb joints and it requires a greater amount of eccentric muscle contraction than walking because of the higher impact forces.[2,5]

The progression of movement of the foot and ankle, knee, hip, pelvis, torso, and upper body will be discussed regarding their role in the running gait cycle.

Stance Phase

The stance phase begins with footstrike, followed by midstance, and then take-off.[4] Different muscle groups, bones, and joints are acting uniquely in each of these actions. At the beginning of foot strike, the muscles, tendons, bones, and joints of the foot and the lower leg function to absorb the impact of the landing.[2,5] The landing during footstrike is facilitated by the actions of the subtalar joint, a multiplanar joint, which causes pronation of the foot. In addition, the plantar fascia stretches to allow the foot to expand and absorb the landing.[6] Dorsiflexion occurs at the level of the talocrural ankle, accompanied by knee flexion, and hip motion, which are all involved in distributing the force of impact through the closed kinetic chain that occurs at footstrike. Rectus femoris and gastrocnemius transfer the energy of impact from

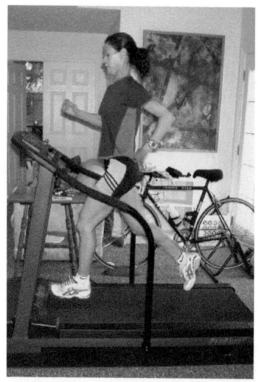

Fig. 3. Swing and stance phases of running. Float phase of the running gait cycle.

distal to proximal (ankle to knee to hip).[7] This helps to distribute the force of the landing, or shock attenuation, throughout the foot and up the kinetic chain. This series of muscle contractions reverses proximal to distal during push off. Incidentally, recent research has found that these kinematics and shock attenuation capability does not change with running-related fatigue of the lower extremity muscles.[8] As the stance phase progresses to midstance, the foot begins to move from pronation to supination in preparation for take-off.[6] The hamstrings shorten and contract as the leg continues through the stance phase.[9] This pulling motion is enhanced by the contraction and push-off motion caused by the gastrocnemius, soleus, and Achilles tendon, which cause plantar flexion of the ankle, and allow for take-off or toe-off. This begins the swing phase. Before discussing the swing phase, we discuss the footstrike in more detail.

There are different patterns of footstrike. One pattern is heelstrike. Most often, the lateral heel strikes the ground as the foot is in supination. The calcaneus is inverted slightly at heelstrike. Additionally, this occurs when the heel strikes the ground first. Midfoot strike is another form of footstrike, which can either occur in heel strike or forefoot strike. Runners who habitually run barefoot land on the forefoot during the running cycle.[10] In contrast, runners who habitually use running shoes tend to land on their heels at footstrike. Pronators land on the outside of the heel and then finish mid to medial forefoot. Supinators will finish stance phase on the lateral forefoot and may not even cause significant heel wear if they are forefoot strikers.

During the running gait cycle, the foot will absorb up to 3 times body weight when striking the ground.[1,11] Running shoes were designed to cushion the foot and allow for neutralization of certain biomechanical differences in runners that were thought to predispose them to injury. However, there is new evidence that suggests that shoes inhibit some adaptive pronation during running gait, which likely protects runners from injury.[12] Shoes, which tend to promote heel strike,[10] have been shown to decrease both metabolic and mechanical efficiency in running.[13] Landing on the midfoot or forefoot during running, typically seen in barefoot runners,[10] helps dissipate impact forces to a greater extent than landing on the heel. This occurs because the foot has a greater degree of plantarflexion at footstrike as well as more compliant ankles.[10] In contrast, running shoe heels can reduce need for ankle dorsiflexion by 5 degrees, allowing for ease of heelstrike. During heelstrike, the ankle is stiffer and unable to distribute impact forces as it would if the footstrike occurred in the midfoot or forefoot.[10] This is because of the inability to translate the impact forces into rotational energy up the kinetic chain through ankle dorsiflexion and knee flexion. This implies as well that barefoot runners who do not adjust their footstrike to midfoot or forefoot strike from heelstrike, will have an increased risk of stress fracture injuries because of the way the impact forces are absorbed.[10] In contrast to the effects of pronation, ground reaction forces that the foot undergoes with running are not affected by the degree of pronation observed in different runners.[14]

Swing Phase

We will now examine the swing phase of the running gait cycle, which occurs when the lower extremity swings through the air from take-off to footstrike. This consists of follow through, forward swing, and foot descent, ending with footstrike which begins the stance phase again.[4] As take-off occurs, rectus femoris and anterior tibialis muscles are the most active.[3] The hamstrings and hip extensors are active during late swing phase.[3] The hamstrings, gastrocsoleus complex, and hip extensors are active from late swing to the middle of the stance phase.[3,15] The float phase includes forward rotation of the ipsilateral pelvis and hip flexion caused by the psoas and other pelvic muscles, along with the core to allow twisting of the pelvis. Rectus femoris is active during the middle of swing phase. The quadriceps begin to show activity during late swing.[3] The hamstrings are lengthening as the lower leg extends at the knee and are most susceptible to injury at the terminal swing.[15] The descent of the foot to the running surface begins. The opposite leg is finishing its stance phase at this time.

Note that in both stance and swing phase, the adductors are active throughout the running gait cycle.

THE KINETIC CHAIN OF RUNNING

As mentioned, the foot and ankle, knee, hip, pelvis, torso, and upper body each play a role in the running gait cycle. To understand the running cycle, one has to have an understanding of the functional anatomy involved in the running gait. Here we review the lower extremity anatomy and the function of various aspects during the running cycle.

The actions of pronation and supination lead to various changes throughout the kinetic chain during the running gait cycle. As pronation occurs, the subtalar joint everts, the forefoot abducts, and the ankle (talocrural) joint dorsiflexes and internally rotates the tibia. The knee follows in a flexed and valgus position. This leads to hip flexion, adduction, and internal rotation. When this occurs, the ipsilateral pelvis rotates anteriorly and elevates to rotate forward on the side of pronation.[2] Finally, the lumbosacral spine extends and lateral flexes ipsilaterally. This series of events along the kinetic chain occur through initial and midstance phase of the running gait cycle.[1,2]

Supination leads to several effects along the kinetic chain as well. As supination occurs, the subtalar joint inverts, the forefoot adducts, the ankle (talocrural) joint plantarflexes, and the tibia externally rotates. At this time, the knee extends into a varus position. This leads to hip extension, abduction, and external rotation. The pelvis rotates posteriorly and depresses on the side of supination. Finally, the lumbosacral joint extends and laterally flexes away from the side of supination.[1,2] This series of events marks the beginning of the swing stage of the running gait cycle.

Foot and Ankle

Running requires the body to absorb continuous repeated impact forces that are initially absorbed by the foot and the ankle and then transferred up the kinetic chain during the stance phase.[16] Each time the foot plants onto the running surface during the running cycle, up to 3 times the weight of the body is absorbed by the lower extremity that lands.[17] The foot must act as a shock absorber, a lever arm to propel the lower extremity forward, and a balance board to keep the body in a straightforward motion, adjusting to uneven running surfaces.

The foot and ankle's ability to do this during the stance phase is facilitated by dorsiflexion, plantarflexion, pronation, and supination.[2,18,19] The actions of pronation and supination play an integral role in the mechanics of the foot and ankle during the running gait cycle. These actions occur at the subtalar joint, which is between the talus and calcaneus.[2,18,19] It is an oblique tarsal joint. This allows the foot and ankle to function efficiently during stance phase running as the impact absorber during pronation and lever arm for propulsion during supination. The subtalar joint axis of the foot follows a 23° (4°– 47° interindividual variation) medially directed and 41° (21°–69°) superiorly directed posterior-to-anterior rotational axis along which subtalar inversion and eversion occur.[2] This orientation allows it to move through the complex range of motions of abduction, adduction, inversion, and eversion that allows pronation and supination of the foot during the running cycle. The calcaneus is about 6 to 8 degrees inverted at footstrike and moves to 6° to 8° of eversion through the rest of stance phase.[1] One study characterized low pronation as 3° to 8.9° of eversion, middle pronation as 9° to 12.9°, and high pronation of 13° to 18° measured while running in shoes.[14] Additionally, Pohl and coworkers[20] reported that eversion of up to about 11° can place abnormal stress on the medial posterior tibia and can be a predictor of a history of tibial stress fracture in runners.

The subtalar joint everts the foot, causing pronation on impact. During pronation, the foot is everted, the forefoot is abducted, and the ankle is dorsiflexed.[1,18,21] The ankle begins dorsiflexion as footstrike occurs.[1,18] This causes internal rotation of the tibia to allow for pronation of the foot.[3] The plantar flexors of the ankle are eccentrically contracting during footstrike to help absorb impact.[2,3,5] Dorsiflexion and pronation at footstrike also facilitate pronation for the purpose of impact absorption.[2] The muscles of plantarflexion also control dorsiflexion during midstance phase of running.[22] They, along with the quadriceps group of muscles, are the main accelerators during the running cycle.[23] The ankle joint is ideally at 90° at footstrike. This progresses to dorsiflexion of 20° from neutral.[2,17] This occurs during midstance as the knee further flexes to absorb the impact of the stance phase. Pronation allows for flexibility in the foot and ankle to accommodate for different running surfaces. The foot is maximally pronated at about halfway through the stance phase.[21] The ligaments in the ankle prevent overpronation, and the tibialis posterior as well as

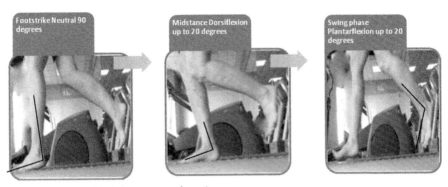

Fig. 4. Running ankle joint ranges of motion.

the gastrocnemius and soleus aid in controlling pronation.[2,6,22] The tibialis anterior muscle has the highest sustained muscle activity in the ankle during the running cycle and likely increases its susceptibility for injury.[22]

The stance phase ends with the foot supinating to create propulsion at toe-off.[3,24] In contrast, supination creates cross alignment of the tarsal joints leading to a stiffer foot and ankle unit and a more efficient lever arm for better propulsion at toe-off during the running cycle.[2] This is, in part, facilitated by the windlass mechanism of the plantar fascia.[2,24] It is also controlled by the posterior tibialis muscle.[3] During supination, the foot is inverted, the forefoot is adducted, and the ankle is plantar-flexed. Because of varying degrees of hindfoot varus and valgus and forefoot varus valgus, each individual has varying degrees of pronation and supination during footstrike and take-off (**Figs. 4** and **5**).

Knee

As mentioned, during pronation, the knee is in valgus position and flexes.[1,2] During supination, it is in varus position and extends.[1,2] It has 2 periods of flexion during the stance and swing phases.[1,3] Knee flexion of 20° to 25° occurs at footstrike and continues to approximately 45° degrees at midstance.[1,3] Flexion at the beginning of stance phase serves as a shock absorber.[3] After footstrike, the quadriceps are active in an eccentric contraction to resist knee flexion.[3] The degree of pronation within the foot tends to impact the degree of knee valgus as well, in that the greater the amount of pronation, the greater the amount of knee valgus within the stance phase.

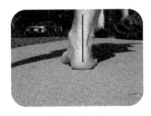
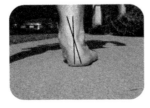
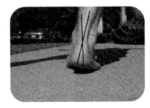

Neutral   Pronation 6-8 degrees at footstrike   Supination 6-8 degrees at toe-off

Fig. 5. Running pronation and supination of the foot.

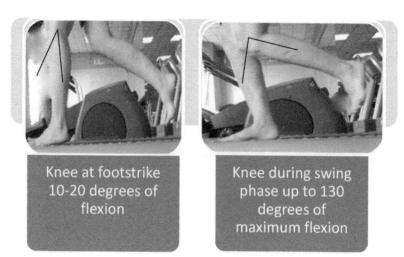

Fig. 6. Running knee joint ranges of motion. Knee flexion range of motion during running gait cycle.

During the swing phase, the knee will maximally flex between 90° and 130° depending on speed.[1,3,25] Minimal power is generated by the muscles crossing the knee during swing phase.[3] Rectus femoris eccentrically contracts to prevent overflexion of the knee in early swing, and then the hamstrings eccentrically contract during late swing to prevent overextension.[3]

The quadriceps group has the primary function of extending the knee. The vastus lateralis, the rectus femoris, the vastus intermedius, and vastus medialis all combine at the superior pole of the patella to extend the knee. Rectus femoris also contributes as a hip flexor during swing. The quadriceps relax at full flexion and then ultimately contract to begin extension of the knee during late swing phase. The knee will extend to within 10° to 20° of full extension.[17] This allows maximum stride length and increases propulsion by increasing the time spent in the air during swing phase. Greater stride lengths increase ground reaction forces at impact, possibly interfering with coordination between the knee and ankle joints and increasing risk of injury (**Fig. 6**).[26]

Hip

Movement of the hip during running gait is to flex during swing and extend during stance phase. The hip adducts during stance phase and abducts during swing phase.[1] The psoas muscle begins swing phase by propelling the thigh forward.[3] The power that the hamstrings and gluteus maximus generate occurs during the second half of the swing phase and the beginning of stance phase. This is when the hamstrings and hip extensors are most active.[3] The abductors and adductors of the hip provide cocontraction stability of the stance leg during single leg support (stance phase). The hip increases flexion range of motion as velocity increases.[3] At footstrike, the hip can be flexed up to 65° in swing phase and extend to 11°.[15] These maximum angles depend on the individual and speed of running. The hamstrings and gluteus maximus extend the hip in the middle of swing phase to "pull" the body forward. The hip will have peak extension at toe-off, which is mostly facilitated by the gluteus maximus.[15] The hip must extend in the late part of swing phase to plant the

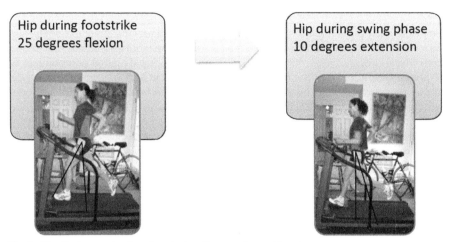

Fig. 7. Hip flexion and extension during the running gait cycle.

foot under center of gravity. This can vary between runners. The hip can go through a full range of about 40° from full flexion to full extension in recreational runners.[25] In the review by Dicharry,[2] hip flexion and extension arc can be as much as 60°. This mainly occurs in the sagittal plane of the body. In addition, the amount of extension in the hip decreases slightly as velocity increases.[17] Hip adductor muscles are active throughout the running gait cycle. This is unique from the walking gait cycle in which they are only active from swing phase to the middle of stance phase.[18] Hip abduction-adduction arc can be as much as 15° (**Fig. 7**).[1]

Pelvis

The pelvis, sacrum, and lumbar vertebrae provide stability to allow the extremities to run. The pelvis relies on symmetry to function during the running cycle. The planes of motion of the pelvis are rotational, anterior-posterior, and medio-lateral. Pelvic biomechanical abnormalities that lead to the most injuries in runners include excessive anterior pelvic tilt, excessive lateral tilt, and asymmetric hip movement. This abnormal pelvic orientation can also lead to excess strain placed on the hamstrings, which can increase rates of injury.[2,27,28] Abnormal pelvic mechanics can also contribute to injury.

Normally, the range of motion of flexion and extension within the pelvis during running is between 5° and 7°.[15] Anterior pelvic tilt is significantly greater during running than in walking, and helps to increase stride length.[29] There is a net 10° to 15° pelvic tilt during running, whereas standing it is about 10°.[15] The degree of pelvic tilt minimally changes with increased velocities of running.[15] In the running cycle, during the single leg stance phase, gluteus medius contracts to keep pelvic tilt stable.[1] At footstrike, the pelvis is posteriorly tilted but still maintains a net anterior tilt approximately 10°. As stance phase begins, the pelvis begins to anteriorly tilt. Maximum anterior tilt occurs immediately after toe-off up to 20°.[15] Abnormal pelvic mechanics, which can influence running gait and lead to overuse injury, can be caused by tight muscles that attach to the pelvis, weakened muscles, or a structural deformity such as scoliosis or a leg length discrepancy.[4]

Torso

The whole body plays a role in the running gait cycle, not just the lower extremity. Hip and lower extremity movement through the running cycle requires a stable and strong core muscle group to allow for motion and limit injury. The dynamic components of the upper torso consist of the ribs, sternum, and thoracic and lumbar vertebrae with supporting ligaments and muscles. The "core" muscles help absorb and distribute impact forces and allow body movements in a controlled and efficient manner. There are 29 core muscles that work together to stabilize the spine, pelvis, and kinetic chain. These consist of the abdominal muscles, paraspinal muscles, gluteal muscles, pelvic floor muscles, hip girdle muscles, and diaphragm.[30] These all work in unison to allow breathing during running and the twisting motion required during the running cycle. Trunk flexion during running is between 3° and 13°.[15] During the running cycle, the trunk is minimally flexed at footstrike and is at its most erect position during the running cycle.[15] It then begins flexion during the stance phase, until maximum flexion occurs at the end of stance phase.[15] Trunk ipsilateral tilt has been measured after foot strike to range from 5° to 20° in coordination with pelvic downward tilt (toward contralateral side). Increasing speed accounted for up to 10° of increase in lateral tilt. As the pelvis rotates each stride, the muscles of the thorax keep the spine and the abdomen stable about the axis of the vertebrae.

Upper Extremities

The arms play a role during the running gait cycle to balance and provide stability to the runner in motion. As a rule, each arm movement counter balances the opposite leg during swing phase. They have also been shown to effectively counterbalance vertical angular momentum during propulsion of the stance phase.[23] Arms aid to balance the torso as well. Arm movement stabilizes the body during running gait cycle and helps the legs run with the most efficiency and least energy expenditure.[31] Lastly, swinging arms assist in the generation of forward momentum during the running cycle.[2,11]

The shoulder joint controls arm movement, and the movement of the legs when strides are taken requires a similar movement of the contralateral arm. The deltoid muscle causes abduction of the arm from the body, which then allows the degrees of movement forward and backward, allowing arm swing about the ball and socket joint of the shoulder. If arm swing is not sufficient, then hip flexion, hip adduction, knee flexion, knee adduction, and ankle abduction have increased joint angles during running cycle (**Fig. 8**).[32]

The pectoral muscles and teres muscles, which attach to the upper humerus, will act with each arm swing to counteract the pull of the deltoid, which actively helps with arm swing. For example, when the left leg swings forward, the right arm swings forward to counter balance the body. Dicharry refers to Novacheck's original description of the arms as a counterbalance for the lower extremities.[1,33] It has been suggested that excessive crossover of the arms is an indicator for the lack of stability of lower body movement; though details of this lack of stability are not specified. The efficiency of running benefits from synchrony of arm and leg swings by minimizing twisting of the torso and pelvis. This saves energy because it allows maximum stride length for the running cycle, and it decreases torso and head rotation.[34]

EVALUATION

There are a number of anatomic variations that are important to consider when assessing a runner who is injured. Evaluation of the runner should include both a

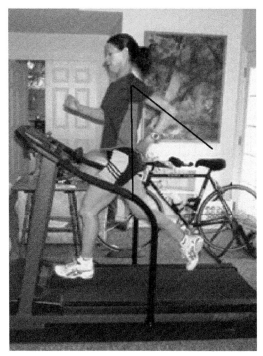

Fig. 8. Arm swing (backward) during running gait cycle.

static and dynamic examination. Examination should include posture as well the entire lower extremity from hips to toes. It should evaluate frontal and transverse planes, extremity length, knee function, ankle dorsiflexion with the knee extended and flexed, configuration of the weight-bearing foot, heel-leg alignment, heel-forefoot alignment, and assessment of footwear. It is important to assess excessive pronation or supination in the runner.[35] Rear foot valgus and rear foot varus occur when the calcaneus is inverted or everted in relation to the bisection of the tibia because of position of the subtalar joint. Forefoot varus and forefoot valgus occur when the forefoot is inverted or everted anterior to the rear foot in the frontal plane.[4] Such foot abnormalities have been associated with plantar fasciitis,[36] sesamoiditis,[4] and stress fractures.[20,37,38]

For example, runners with pronated feet during the stance phase will more often have sesamoiditis, plantar fasciitis, Achilles tendinopathy, medial shin pain, patellar tendinopathy, patellofemoral pain, metatarsal stress fractures, navicular stress fractures, and fibular stress fractures.[4,21] The gastrocnemius and soleus and tibialis posterior muscle overcompensate for the excessive internal rotation of the lower extremity in overpronators. Each contracts longer to stop the internal rotation of the tibia caused by the excessive pronation. This can lead to Achilles tendinopathy and tibialis posterior tendinopathy and can contribute to medial shin pain caused by excessive forces placed on the medial tibia.[4,39] Alignment can be affected by excessive pronation as well. The increased internal rotation of the lower leg can lead to lateral patellar subluxation and quadriceps muscle firing imbalance, which are the hallmarks of patellofemoral pain syndrome. Also, a foot that overpronates tends to cause uneven distribution of the force of impact to the medial tibia and knee.

Table 1
Common biomechanical abnormalities and associated injuries

Injury	Pelvis	Hip	Knee	Ankle	Foot
IT band syndrome	Increased anterior or posterior tilt[4,15]	Increased hip adduction[42] Femoral neck anteversion[36]	Genu varum[4]		
Posterior tibial tendonopathy					Hyper/hypo- pronation[36]
Hamstring strain	Excessive anterior pelvic tilt[1,27,28]			Ankle equines[4]	
Medial/lateral/anterior compartment syndrome			Patella alta[36]		
Flexor hallicis longus tendonitis					Cavus foot/flat foot[36]
Patellofemoral pain	Anterior pelvic tilt[4]	Weak hip abductors[41]	Excessive Q angle,[36] Genu Varum[4]		Overpronation[4]
Stress fractures		Increased hip adduction[20,37]	Squinting patella,[36] hypermobile patella,[36] Genu varum[4]		Hindfoot varus,[20,37,38] oversupination,[4] overpronation[4]
Achilles tendinopathy			External tibial torsion[36]	Ankle equines[4]	Overpronation[4]
Sesamoiditis					Overpronation,[4] forefoot valgus[4]
Low back pain	Anterior pelvic tilt[1,40]	Leg length discrepancy[36]			
Medial tibial stress syndrome					Overpronation[39]
Plantar fasciitis					Forefoot valgus/varus,[36] overpronation,[4] oversupination,[4] ankle equines[4]
Sacroiliac dysfunction	Increased pelvic rotation[15]				
Patellar tendonitis	Anterior pelvic tilt[4]		Genu varum[4,36] Genu valgum[36]		Overpronation[4]
Peroneal tendiopathy					Oversupination[4]

Conditions that cause knee pain in runners can be caused by femoral neck anteversion, genu varum, squinting patellae, excessive q angle, tibia varum, functional equines, and pronated feet. An individual with an abnormal or inefficient running action is more likely to suffer injury than someone with good mechanics. In addition, an individual with anatomy that deviates from the "normal" can sometimes have a higher rate of injuries as well.

Runners with excessive supination tend to have poor mobility and fail to absorb the impact of footstrike. Excessive supination can occur at the subtalar joint, often in compensation for abnormal foot anatomy or musculature (such as high arches or peroneal muscle weakness). More force distributed through the lateral aspect of the foot in supinated runners will lead to peroneal tendinopathy, metatarsal stress fractures, and fibular stress fractures more often than a neutral foot.[4] There is also poor control of the lateral muscles of the foot and ankle. In addition, feet with high arches tend to not be able to distribute this force as evenly, as the lateral aspect of the foot absorbs the majority of the impact of the landing of footstrike.

With regard to lumbopelvic dynamic deficits, excessive anterior pelvic tilt is mostly caused by stretched and weak gluteal muscles. This inability to contract evenly or strongly can lead to an unstable pelvis during the running gait cycle as well as contribute to increased lateral tilt.[4] Excessive lateral tilt can also be caused by weakness or inflexibility in the adductor or abductor muscle groups of the hip. This can lead to inability of the hip to maintain a normal forward plane of motion. Also, the opposite hip has greater difficulty dropping and rotating during its swing phase. Pelvic asymmetry can be caused by tight muscles within the pelvis and core or structural abnormalities, such as leg length discrepancy or scoliosis. When pelvic asymmetry is present and uncorrected, running will more than likely lead to overuse injuries, which can improve if the pelvic asymmetry is corrected.[4]

KINETIC CHAIN

Finally, if the hip has increased mobility, there will be an increased movement of the ipsilateral knee, contralateral hip, and the lumbar spine to compensate. Limited hip flexor mobility can shift pelvic orientation anteriorly and may place the lumbar spine in a nonneutral position and lead to low back pain.[1,40] This will cause strain in the hamstrings as well. In addition, weakness in hip abductors leads to conditions such as patellofemoral pain syndrome.[41] Certain structural and biomechanical deviations from the norm in runners can and will lead to specific types of injuries. **Table 1** summarizes the biomechanical abnormalities that can lead to various overuse injuries in runners.

SUMMARY

To understand the normal series of biomechanical events of running, a comparative assessment to walking is helpful. Closed kinetic chain through the lower extremities, control of the lumbopelvic mechanism, and overall symmetry of movement has been described well enough that deviations from normal movement can now be associated with specific overuse injuries experienced by runners. This information in combination with a history of the runner's errors in their training program will lead to a more comprehensive treatment and prevention plan for related injuries.

REFERENCES

1. Dicharry J. Kinematics and kinetics of gait: from lab to clinic. Clin Sports Med 2010;29(3):347–64.

2. Dugan S, Bhat K. Biomechanics and analysis of running gait. Phys Med Rehabil Clin North Am 2005;16(3):603–21.

3. Novacheck TF. The biomechanics of running. Gait Posture 1998;7:77–95.

4. Brukner P, Khan K. Biomechanics of Common Sporting Injuries. In: Clinical sports medicine. 3rd edition. Sydney (Australia): McGraw-Hill; 2008. p. 40–61.

5. Ounpuu S. The biomechanics of walking and running. Clin Sport Med 1994;13(4): 843–63.

6. Perry J. Anatomy and biomechanics of the hindfoot. Clin Orthop Relat Res 1983; (177): 9–15.

7. Prilutsky B, Zatsiorsky V. Tendon action of two-joint muscles: transfer of mechanical energy between joints during jumping, landing, and running. J Biomech 1994;27(1): 25–34.

8. Abt J, Sell T, Chu Y, et al. Running kinematics and shock absorption do not change after brief exhaustive running. J Strength Cond Res 2011;25(6):1479–85.

9. Tweed J, Campbell J, Avil S. Biomechanical risk factors in the development of medial tibial stress syndrome in distance runners. J Am Podiatr Med Assoc 2008;98(6):436–44.

10. Lieberman D, Madhusudhan V, Werbel W, et al. Foot strike patterns and collision forces in habitually barefoot versus shod runners. Nature 2010;463:531–5.

11. Mann RA Biomechanics of running. In: Mack RP, editor. American Academy of Orthopaedic Surgeons Symposium on the Foot and Leg in Running Sports. St Louis (MO): C.V. Mosby; 1982. p.1–29.

12. Vormittag K, Calonje R, Briner WW. Foot and ankle injuries in the barefoot sports. Curr Sports Med Rep 2009;8(5):262–6.

13. Prilutsky B, Zatsiorsky V. Tendon action of two-joint muscles: transfer of mechanical energy between joints during jumping, landing, and running. J Biomech 1994;27(1): 25–34.

14. Morley J, Decker L, Dierks T, et al. Effects of varying amounts of pronation on the medial ground reaction forces during barefoot versus shod running. J Appl Biomech 2010;26(2):205–14.

15. Schache A, Bennell K, Blanch P, et al. The coordinated movement of the lumbo-pelvic-hip complex during running: a literature review. Gait and Posture 1999;10:30–47.

16. Donatelli RA. Normal biomechanics of the foot and ankle. J Orthop Sports Phys Ther 1985;7(3):91–5.

17. James SL, Jones, DC. Biomechanical aspects of distance running injuries. In: Cavanaugh PR, editor. Biomechanics of distance running. Champaign (IL): Human Kinetics Books; 1990. p. 249–70.

18. Mann R, Hagy J. Biomechanics of walking, running, and sprinting. Am J Sports Med 1980;8:345.

19. James S, Bates B, Ostering L. Injuries to runners. Am J Sports Med 1978;6(2):40–50.

20. Pohl M, Mullineaux D, Milner C, et al. Biomechanical predictors of retrospective tibial stress fractures in runners. J Biomech 2008;41(6):1160–5.

21. Sinning W, Forsyth H. Lower-limb actions while running at different velocities. Med Sci Sports 1970;2:28–34.

22. Reber L, Perry J, Pink M. Muscular control of the ankle in running. Am J Sports Med 1993;21(6):805–10.

23. Hamner S, Seth A, Delp S. Muscle contributions to propulsion and support during running. J Biomech 2010;43(14):2709–16.

24. Hockenbury R. Forefoot problems in athletes. Med Sci Sports Exerc 1999;31(7 Suppl):s448–58.

25. Pink M, Perry J, Houglum P, et al. Lower extremity range of motion in the recreational sport runner. Am J Sports Med 1994;22(4):541–9.
26. Stergiou N, Bates BT, Kurz MJ. Subtalar and knee joint interaction during running at various stride lengths. J Sports Med Phys Fitness 2003;43(3):319–26.
27. Chumanov E, Heiderscheit B, Thelen D. The effect of speed and influence of individual muscles on hamstring mechanics during the swing phase of sprinting. J Biomech 2007;40(16):3555–62.
28. Thelen D, Chumanov E, Sherry M, et al. Neuromusculoskeletal models provide insights into the mechanisms and rehabilitation of hamstring strains. Exerc Sport Sci Rev 2006;34(3):135–41.
29. Williams KR. Biomechanics of running. Exerc Sport Sci Rev 1985;13:389–441.
30. Elliott B, Blanksby B. A biomechanical analysis of the male jogging action. J Human Move Stud 1979:5;42–51.
31. Arellano CJ, Kram R. The effects of step width and arm swing on energetic cost and lateral balance during running. J Biomech 2011;29:44(7):1291–5.
32. Miller R, Caldwell G, Van Emmerik R, et al. Ground reaction forces and lower extremity kinematics when running with suppressed arm swing. J Biomech Eng 2009;131(12):121–5.
33. Novacheck TF, Trost JP, Schutte L. Running and sprinting: a dynamic analysis. St Paul (MN): Gillette Children's Hospital; 1996. [Video CD-ROM].
34. Pontzer H, Holloway J, Raichlen D, et al. Control and function of arm swing in human walking and running. J Exp Biol 2009;212(Pt 4):523–34.
35. Plastaras C, Rittenberg J, Rittenberg K, et al. Comprehensive functional evaluation of the injured runner. Phys Med Rehabil Clin North Am 2005;16:623–49.
36. Kannus V. Evaluation of abnormal biomechanics of the foot and ankle in athletes. Br J Sp Med 1992;26(2):83–9.
37. Milner C, Hamill J, Davis I. Distinct hip and rearfoot kinematics in female runners with a history of tibial stress fracture. J Orthop Sports Phys Ther 2010;40(2):59–66.
38. Pohl M, Mullineaux D, Milner C, et al. Biomechanical predictors of retrospective tibial stress fractures in runners. J Biomech 2008;41(6):1160–5.
39. Tweed J, Campbell J, Avil S. Biomechanical risk factors in the development of medial tibial stress syndrome in distance runners. J Am Podiatr Med Assoc 2008;98(6):436–44.
40. Hodges PW. Core stability exercise in chronic low back pain. Orthop Clin North Am 2003;34(2):245–54.
41. Dierks TA, Manal KT, Hamill J, et al. Proximal and distal influences on hip and knee kinematics in runners with patellofemoral pain during a long run. J Orthop Sports Phys Ther 2008;38(8):448–56.
42. Ferber R, Noehren B, Hamill J, et al. Competitive female runners with a history of iliotibial band syndrome demonstrate atypical hip and knee kinematics. J Orthop Sports Phys Ther 2010;40(2):52–8.

Evaluation of the Injured Runner

Alexander K. Meininger, MD[a],*, Jason L. Koh, MD[b]

KEYWORDS

- Physical examination • Running • Injury • Overuse
- Tendinitis

HISTORY

Evaluation of the injured runner begins with a thorough history. The goal is to understand the nature of the pain, identify risk factors, and facilitate a trustworthy relationship with the athlete. Often, the runner will have sought other opinions or received diagnoses before presentation. Researching their symptoms and self-diagnosing is also commonplace with the widespread dissemination of medical knowledge online. Understanding any preconceived notions is important before delivering diagnoses and recommending treatment.

The medical history is the first step toward developing a productive patient relationship. Clarifying the athlete's pain complaints and mechanism of injury is the first goal. Standard questions regarding location, duration, onset, course, quality, and intensity as well as exacerbating and ameliorating factors guide the encounter (**Table 1**). Does the pain occur only with activity? Or is there pain at rest? When does the pain begin—at the outset of a run or game, in the middle, or near the end? Has this pain ever occurred before? Determine what evaluations and investigations have already been performed. Has your runner seen anyone else for this problem—an athletic trainer, physical therapist, chiropractor, or physician? What diagnoses or treatments were given? Previous therapies and their effectiveness should be reviewed. Does the pain improve with massage, bracing, or anti-inflammatories? If a period of rest has been undertaken, clarify the details. How many weeks were spent away from running? What type of cross training was used? Did the symptoms resolve or recur?

A complete history should also disclose facets such as developmental abnormalities, potentially confounding medical issues, and prior surgical procedures. Medications,

Dr Meininger has no disclosures.

[a] Orthopaedic Surgery & Sports Medicine, Moab Regional Specialty Clinic, 476 West Williams Way, Suite B, Moab, UT 84532, USA

[b] Department of Orthopaedic Surgery, North Shore University Health System, 1000 Central Street, Suite 880, Evanston, IL 60201, USA

* Corresponding author.

E-mail address: meininga@gmail.com

Clin Sports Med 31 (2012) 203–215

doi:10.1016/j.csm.2011.11.002

0278-5919/12/$ – see front matter © 2012 Elsevier Inc. All rights reserved.

sportsmed.theclinics.com

Table 1 Varied clinical presentations and common diagnoses for leg pain in the running athlete	
Was there an acute onset of pain?	Fractures and tendon ruptures are usually acute traumatic events. In athletes, the acute onset of pain may be preceded by low-grade chronic pain of a stress fracture or tendinosis.
Is there a history of injury, surgery, or pain?	Old injury may predispose to scarring, stiffness, or pain.
Is the pain worsened with exertion?	Pain absent at rest that presents with exertion is characteristic of exertional compartment syndrome.
Does the pain improve with warm-up and stretching?	Muscle strains and medial tibial stress syndrome frequently will improve.
Is there electrical, shooting pain, weakness or numbness?	Radiating pain, dermatomal loss of sensation, or root-specific weakness may indicate nerve injury, entrapment, or radiculopathy. Always check the lumbar spine.

supplements, or performance-enhancing drugs are important to the treating clinician. For instance, a history of corticosteroid use may increase the risk for stress fractures,[1] whereas creatine monohydrate supplements may increase intracompartmental muscle pressures through increased intracellular fluid.[2] Dietary habits and nutrition, including dairy and calcium intake, should also be discussed.

The injured female runner deserves special mention here. The highest risk for stress fracture is a history of prior stress fractures.[3] Risk factors for stress fracture, including eating disorders, amenorrhea, and osteopenia, are considered the "female athlete triad." Menstrual history, including age at menarche, regularity, and date of last period are important queries. Additionally, consideration should be given to anatomic differences, such as wider pelvic width, increased foot pronation, and decreased body mass index that may place women at increased risk for injury, including stress fracture.[4–6]

Outlining a runner's training habits is the second goal of a complete history. Errors in training are the most common causes, and injuries often result when runners undertake "too much, too soon."[7] Training regimens including weekly mileage and intensity can help identify predisposing factors. Abrupt changes in running frequency, mileage increases, transitioning from indoors to outdoors, or abruptly adding hill or interval workouts can increase the strain on the musculoskeletal system.[8] Goals and aspirations ought to be discussed as well. For instance, the recreational runner in pursuit of his or her first marathon may present with different issues than the seasoned track athlete in competition. Practitioners may find a detailed patient intake questionnaire helpful to summarize a runner's habits (**Fig. 1**).[7]

PHYSICAL EXAMINATION

Physical examination of the injured runner should be both focused and comprehensive. Goals of evaluation are not only to discern the local sources of pain, but also to identify biomechanical risk factors and functional limitations predisposing to injury. A sequence or flow to the physical examination that is repeated easily is the best method to ensure nothing is missed. Our technique as described below is efficient and reproducible in any outpatient setting.

RUNNER'S EVALUATION FORM

Training History

Level of Competition:
- ☐ Recreational only
- ☐ Recreational competitive
- ☐ Competitive (HS/college)
- ☐ Elite

Running Surface:
- ☐ Treadmill
- ☐ Street (asphalt)
- ☐ Sidewalk (concrete)
- ☐ Trail
- ☐ Track

Cross-Training:
- ☐ Biking
- ☐ Swimming
- ☐ Weights
- ☐ Stairs
- ☐ Yoga/Stretching
- ☐ Other:

Years of running: _____
Running Club: _____
Pace/mile: _____
Mileage/week: _____
Long run: _____
Runs/week: _____
Shoe type: _____
Miles on shoe: _____

Shoe Insert or Orthotics: ☐ Yes ☐ No
Are you in training?:   ☐ Yes ☐ No   *Race and Date:* _____

Recent change in your training ?
- ☐ Increased mileage
- ☐ New shoes or inserts
- ☐ Speed work or track work
- ☐ Hill training
- ☐ Change in terrain

When you run. when do symptoms occur?
- ☐ Every step of the run
- ☐ Worse toward the end of the run
- ☐ Worse at start & then improves
- ☐ Only after the run ends (next day)

Medical History

Date and Description of Injury: _____
Previous Treatments for Injury: _____
Past Medical & Surgical History: _____
Medications: _____
Allergies: _____
Prior Musculoskeletal Injuries: _____

History of stress fractures: ☐ Yes ☐ No
    steroid use: ☐ Yes ☐ No
    osteoporosis: ☐ Yes ☐ No
    eating disorders: ☐ Yes ☐ No

Female History: ☐ N/A
    reg. periods: ☐ Yes ☐ No
    pregnant: ☐ Yes ☐ No
    age of 1st period: _____
    date of last period: _____

Fig. 1. Runner's evaluation intake sheet. (*From* Plastaras CT, Rittenberg JD, Rittenberg KE, et al. Comprehensive functional evaluation of the injured runner. Phys Med Rehabil Clin North Am 2005;16(3):623–49; with permission.)

Site-Specific Examination

Our examination begins with a direct assessment of the runner's primary complaint. With the patient seated on the examination table, the affected limb is observed for swelling, ecchymoses, or discoloration. Redness and swelling of the tibia, calcaneus, or midfoot can be of a sign of underlying stress fracture or acute injury. Both feet are inspected for "hot spots," calluses, or blisters. Prominence of the calcaneal tuberosity is known as *Haglund's deformity*. Its association with shoe pressure has led to the common description of a "pump bump." Forefoot deformities, such as bunions, hammer toes, and claw toes should be recognized. Thickened or cornified skin on the dorsum of the interphalangeal joints or dark nail discoloration (as occurs with a subungal hematoma) may reflect recurrent friction or injury. Each may be an indirect sign of poor-fitting or worn out footwear.

Subsequently, a thorough palpation examination is begun distant to the point of maximal tenderness. The astute examiner may appreciate discrete soft tissue swelling, fullness, or crepitations in areas of tendinopathy or stress reaction. Percussion of bony prominences (such as Gerdy's tubercle, the anterior tibial crest, medial and lateral malleoli, and dorsal metatarsals) will also help uncover symptoms of stress reaction.[9] Pain elicited with palpation, or a "squeeze test," of the calcaneus or midfoot can signify stress reaction or ligamentous injury.[10] Pain with application of a 128-Hz tuning fork is highly sensitive for stress injury. Fascial defects and muscle herniations often are readily palpable in the leg. A Tinel's sign may be elicited in cases of nerve entrapment or Morton's neuroma. In addition, circulation, sensation, and reflexes can be checked at this time.

Motion and strength of the foot and ankle are assessed next. Passive subtalar eversion and inversion should approximate 20° and 40°, respectively.[11] Decreased subtalar motion and forefoot pronation is associated with increased overuse injuries in runners. Active inversion is tested in the figure-4 position with the athlete directing the forefoot toward the ceiling (**Fig. 2**). Pain with resistance may be associated with posterior tibial tendinitis.

Asking the runner to point his or her toes as far as possible tests plantarflexion. Normal plantarflexion approximates 50°. Loss of plantarflexion may be caused by posterior ankle impingement or an os trigonum. Passive dorsiflexion of the ankle is performed while inverting the forefoot with a neutral hindfoot. This technique locks the midtarsal joints and provides a more accurate assessment of true sagittal ankle motion. Normal ankle dorsiflexion averages 20°. Runners with diminished dorsiflexion

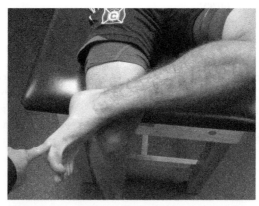

Fig. 2. Clinical photograph of inversion strength testing using the **Fig. 4** position.

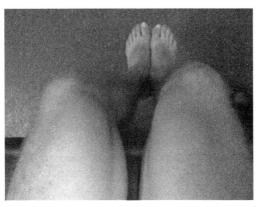

Fig. 3. Clinical photograph of the bilateral flexed knees with increased lateral patellar tilt.

commonly have a tight gastrocsoleus complex. Testing dorsiflexion in both straight and flexed positions can help to discern if tightness is originating from the gastrocnemius or soleus portions. Dorsiflexion that worsens with knee extension indicates an isolated contracture of the gastrocnemius.

Examination of the knee should also begin in the seated position. Resting patellar tilt is easily recognized with the knee bent 90° (**Fig. 3**). Flexion makes taut the patellar tendon facilitating direct palpation. Pain or crepitus at the distal patellar pole may be a sign of patellar tendinitis. Tenderness or prominence of the tibial tubercle in the skeletally immature may be a sign of traction apophysitis at the tibial tubercle (Osgood-Schlatter's disease) or distal patella (Sinding-Larsen-Johannsen syndrome). Patellar tracking and crepitations are evaluated dynamically, as the patient is asked to straighten the knee from 90° of flexion to full extension. Maltracking often manifests with a positive "J sign" in which the patella abruptly deviates laterally once it disengages from the femoral trochlea. Lastly, the seated straight leg raise and slump test for neural tension signs are easily performed at this time.

Supine Examination

The remainder of the knee examination takes place with the runner supine. Swelling or fullness about the knee can be caused by intra-articular fluid or extra-articular soft tissue swelling. An effusion can be recognized with the fluid wave test, where the examiner "milks" the knee from the suprapatellar pouch distally while palpating for fluid in the parapatellar hollows with the other hand. The patellofemoral joint is evaluated for pain with compression (patellar chondromalacia or osteoarthritis) and lateral tightness with tilt testing (lateral patellar compression syndrome). Range of motion is assessed first with the examiner raising both feet in the air. Symmetric knee extension should allow the knees to fall at the same level with the patient relaxed. Normal knees may hyperextend 5° to 10°. Flexion is assessed by bending the knee as far as possible. Normal range is 130° to 150° depending on body habitus and can easily be compared with the heel-buttock distance. A standard examination is then performed for ligamentous laxity or meniscal pathology.

Straight hip flexion, rotation, and abduction are also assessed supine. Adduction and extension are best tested with the patient lying on his or her side (see below). Normal flexion is 110° to 120°, internal rotation 30° to 40°, external rotation 40° to 60°, and abduction 30° to 50°. Pain with impingement testing, or combined flexion, adduction, and internal rotation, is highly suggestive of an acetabular labral tear.[12] Hamstring flexibility is assessed with the hips flexed 90° and the knee extended until resistance is encountered. The popliteal angle is acute angle subtended by the tibial and femoral axes.

Special tests for the hip and pelvis are also useful. The Thomas test is valuable to assess length of the iliopsoas and tensor fascia lata. Tight hip flexors are a common complaint in runners. The patient flexes both hips against the chest to stabilize the pelvis, and then the examiner extends the hip to be tested while the opposite knee is held against the chest. If the thigh is unable to reach the examination table, a flexion contracture is present. The flexion-abduction-external rotation (or FABER) test stresses the sacroiliac joint and anterior hip. It is performed with the limb in the figure-4 position with downward pressure applied to the ipsilateral knee while stabilizing the pelvis.

Side Lying Examination

This position affords excellent access to the lateral hip. Tenderness about the greater trochanter can be reproduced easily with deep palpation. Additionally, the Noble test for iliotibial band (ITB) tightness can be performed with compression of the ITB proximal to the knee joint. Flexibility of the ITB is measured with the Ober test.[13] In this test, the examiner stands behind the patient and stabilizes the pelvis. The hip is abducted 30°, the knee is flexed 90°, and passive adduction is observed. Normal flexibility should allow for 20° of cross-limb adduction. Diminished range, as is common in runners, is a sign of a tight ITB. Open chain abduction strength can be assessed with the hip held in neutral flexion and slight external rotation against resistance. Subtle deficiencies in abductor strength may not manifest until dynamic testing is performed (see below). Hip flexibility is examined next. Normal hip extension is 10° to 30° (**Fig. 4**).

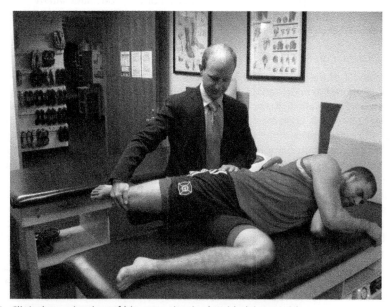

Fig. 4. Clinical examination of hip extension in the side-lying position.

Prone Examination

The prone position affords further evaluation of the athlete's flexibility, lower extremity alignment. Flexibility of the rectus femoris is tested with the Ely test. In the prone position, the knee is passively flexed beyond 90°. Associated hip flexion or lifting the ipsilateral pelvis from the examination table is a positive result. Additionally, a femoral nerve tension test can be performed with passive knee flexion and hip extension in the prone position. Dural tension is aggravated in this position and relieved on relaxation. Ankle dorsiflexion may also be evaluated prone. Normal range is 10°. Femoral anteversion can be assessed clinically by flexing the knee 90° while internally rotating the hip. When the greater trochanter becomes palpable, the angle subtended by the long axis of the tibia from the vertical represents the femoral anteversion.

Standing Examination

The standing examination is invaluable for assessment of spinal, pelvic and lower extremity alignment. In double limb weight bearing the athlete is observed in 3 planes. The examiner begins by viewing the patient from behind. Shoulder droop, prominent scapula, or pelvic tilt may be subtle signs of scoliosis. Lateral bending ought to be symmetric and segmental dysfunction noted. Spinal range of motion is tested in flexion by asking the patient to bend at the waist and touch his or her toes. Simultaneous palpation of the posterior superior iliac spines allows for assessment of the sacroiliac joints. Pain with spinal extension may signify stress injury of the posterior spine or spondylolysis. The most sensitive examination for spondylolysis is the single-leg hyperextension test, or flamingo test. The patient is asked to stand on 1 foot, and pain elicited with lumbar spinal hyperextension is a positive sign. Pelvic obliquity is evaluated with the examiner's hands palpating the iliac crests and anterior and posterior iliac spines. Abnormal tilt may be a sign of scoliosis, sacroiliac joint dysfunction, or limb length discrepancy.

Lower extremity alignment is also observed standing. Genu varum is common in men and genu valgum in women. Both remain physiologic within 5° of neutral. Patellae face forward in the normal resting alignment. Excessive internal rotation or "squinting patellae" may predispose to patellofemoral syndrome. The quadriceps angle, or Q-angle, is the intersection of a line drawn from the anterior superior iliac spine to the midpatella and another line from the midpatella to the tibial tubercle.[14] Normal is 10° in men and 15° in women. Excessive Q-angles have been associated with patellar maltracking and patellofemoral pain syndromes.[15] The "miserable malalignment" syndrome is a constellation of findings common in female runners complaining of anterior knee pain. It is characterized by an excessive Q-angle, increased femoral anteversion, relative tibial external rotation, and foot pronation.

The feet are observed for pes planus or pes cavus. Pes planus is a flexible pronated foot with loss of the medial longitudinal arch. Excessive foot pronation is commonly associated with running overuse injuries, including medial tibial stress syndrome, exertional compartment syndrome, stress fractures, and tendonopathies. Arch height can be evaluated clinically with the navicular drop test, although its reliability remains in question.[16] In this test, the height of the navicular is measured while standing in both the subtalar neutral and relaxed positions.[17] A loss in height greater than 1.5 cm is considered abnormal and an indication for dynamic stability control training and foot orthoses.

The cavus foot has a plantarflexed first ray and an inverted hindfoot, causing a high arch (**Fig. 5**). The forefoot is more rigid with less motion. Diminished flexibility results

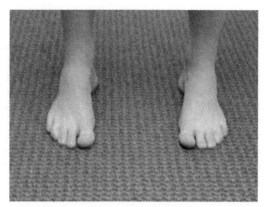

Fig. 5. Clinical photograph of cavus feet. (*From* Desai SN, Grierson R, Manoli A. The cavus foot in athletes: fundamentals of examination and treatment. Oper Tech Sports Med 2010;18:27–33; with permission.)

in decreased force, dampening and increasing stress on the foot, ankle, and leg. However, in one study of 449 Naval recruits, both pes planus and pes cavus were found to be risk factors for lower extremity overuse injuries.[18] A less-rigid orthotic helps support the foot and improve shock absorption.

GAIT

Gait analysis is critical in the evaluation of the injured runner. In the clinical setting, a screening walking examination can be performed easily. Because we begin our encounter with the site of injury, our gait evaluation logically follows the standing examination.

Patients are asked to walk at a casual pace without shoes or socks. The examiner observes the athlete from the front, side, and behind. Attention is immediately given to asymmetries in joint motion, stride length, or duration of single leg stance, such as occur with contractures, limb length inequalities, or an antalgic gait. The foot and ankle are observed for heel strike and foot pronation with initial contact and loading. Athletes are then asked to toe walk and heel walk. Toe walking demonstrates plantarflexion range of motion, gastrocsoleus, and posterior tibialis strength. Heel walking accentuates tibialis anterior dorsiflexion weakness.

Advanced techniques of treadmill testing may also be performed, although these may require additional time, staff, or resources. Similarly, provocative testing with running or stair climbing may be necessary to elicit exercise-induced leg pain, such as exertional compartment syndrome. Coordination with an allied health professional, such as a physical therapist or certified athletic trainer, may help facilitate these modalities.

Formal gait analysis with high-speed cinematography, electromyography, kinetic force plates, and infrared cameras is available in some centers. Reflective markers are placed on anatomic landmarks to define limb axes. Data are digitized by computer, and joint motion during phases of the gait cycle can be defined. Commercialization of the technology has led to the widespread use of electronic gait analysis in specialist running and sports shops. However, their effectiveness remains unproven.

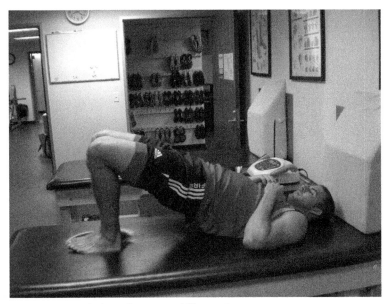

Fig. 6. Pelvic bridge technique for core stability testing.

CORE STABILITY AND BALANCE

Functional testing challenges the core musculature and may identify strength deficits not obvious in the prior examination. The pelvic bridge test recruits the gluteals, hamstrings, paraspinal, and abdominal muscles. While supine, the athlete places the feet flat on the examination table with the knees flexed and lifts the pelvis toward the ceiling (**Fig. 6**). Inability to hold the position or hamstring cramping signals gluteus maximus weakness.[7] Unilateral leg raises in the bridge position may identify side-to-side differences indicative of pelvic floor and hip abductor weakness.

The single-leg squat is a reliable predictor of hip abductor strength that has been validated in the clinical setting with good interrater reliability ($\kappa = 0.80$).[19,20] Athletes are asked to perform a single-leg squat, lowering themselves as far as possible and returning to standing without losing balance. A Trendelenburg sign (a contralateral dip in the pelvic frontal plane) may manifest once the athlete assumes single leg stance. Weak hip abductors will cause excessive hip adduction, internal rotation, and a lack of knee control, or "wobble." Poor trunk control and excessive hip internal rotation have been shown to put female athletes at risk for hip and knee injury.[19,20]

Provocative testing may also be useful to discern subtle strength imbalances. Both double- and single-leg vertical jumps can be performed, although single-leg jumps have been shown to better define unilateral strength imbalances.[21] Single-leg hopping is also used as a provocative test in cases of clinical suspicion for bony pathology or stress fractures.

Although the double- and single-leg vertical jumps require the use of portable force plates for power measurement, a more convenient clinical assessment may be the 5-hop test as described by Newton.[21] Subjects begin on 2 feet, hop forward onto 1 foot, and then perform 4 consecutive hops on 1 leg, landing with both feet on the fifth hop. Athletes attempt to maximize the longitudinal distance covered (measured in centimeters). Three trials are performed for each the right and left legs. Reliability was

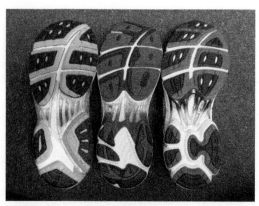

Fig. 7. Pictured (*left to right*): straight, semicurved and curved last running shoes. Note the increasing curvature of the soles from heel to toe.

high with an intraclass correlation of 0.892, and statistically significant differences were detected between dominant and nondominant lower extremities in their study. Clearly, simple testing with the single-leg vertical jump or 5-hop test can quickly determine unilateral strength deficits.

Shoewear

Lastly, it is important not to overlook the runner's footwear. Runners should have both current and previous shoes available during their visit. The age and mileage on the shoes should be determined. In general, running shoes tend to deteriorate after 300 to 500 miles and should be replaced annually or sooner as mileage dictates. Shock-absorbing shoes with cushioned midsoles may wear more quickly especially in extreme heat or wet surfaces.

Patterns of wear and shoe shape offer clues toward fit and alignment. Normally, some wear in the lateral heel occurs at initial contact. However, excessive lateral forefoot wear may signify a cavus foot and supinated gait. Medial forefoot wear, on the other hand, is associated with excessive pronation.

Not all shoes are meant to fit all foot types. The last, or shape of the shoe, may be straight, curved, or semicurved (**Fig. 7**). A curved last offers a lighter, more flexible shoe, commonly found in track spikes. Flexibility is also ideal for the high arched or cavus foot. Straight last shoes carry the moniker "motion control shoes" because they are stiffer from heel to toe with additional medial arch support for pronated flat feet (**Fig. 8**). However, a recent study by Ryan and colleagues[22] disputed this claim. Eighty-one female runners participating in a 13-week half-marathon training program were grouped by foot type (neutral, pronated, highly pronated) and randomly assigned running shoes (neutral, stability, and motion control). Surprisingly, the group of highly pronated feet assigned to the motion control shoes reported the most missed training days because of running-related leg pain. Conversely, relatively few missed training days were reported in the highly pronated runners with neutral shoes. Clearly, footwear plays a role in the biomechanics of running. However, further research is necessary to determine the most appropriate shoe for each foot type.

Barefoot running has increased in popularity and gained attention of the press.[23] Advocates argue barefoot running is more natural, has been practiced for millions of

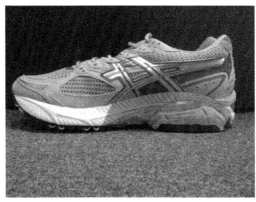

Fig. 8. Motion control straight last shoes marketed toward runners with pronated feet. Note the increased medial arch support.

years, and has yielded success at the elite level since the 1960s.[24] Biomechanical and gait studies have found decreased stride length, increased cadence, and increased ankle plantarflexion at initial contact.[25,26] Robbins and Hanna[27] found these gait alterations allowed for initial contact at the metatarsal heads, facilitating intrinsic foot muscle strengthening and maintenance of the longitudinal arch. The investigators suggest these adaptations reduce the impact of running and decrease the risk of injury.[25]

Disadvantages of barefoot running include the risk of blunt or penetrating trauma, thermal or frostbite injury, and the potential for increased shock on impact.[28] Barefoot-simulating footwear has been developed in an attempt to reduce these risks and has reliably reproduced barefoot running biomechanics.[26] Essentially consisting of a sole and upper, the Vibram FiveFingers (Vibram, Concord, MA, USA) (**Fig. 9**) is one example. A recent report including 2 metatarsal stress injuries in experienced runners after transitioning to barefoot-simulated running highlights the risks involved.[29] The clinical evidence supporting or rejecting barefoot running, however, is only anecdotal at present.[30]

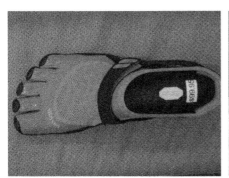
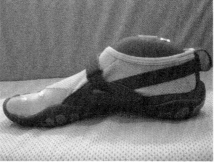

Fig. 9. Vibram® FiveFingers is one popular example of barefoot-simulating footwear.

SUMMARY

Leg pain in runners is a common complaint in any sports medicine practice. Although the possible diagnoses are many, the evaluation depends on a thorough history. A comprehensive physical examination should include not only examination of the injury but the kinetic chain and core. It is imperative to recognize functional deficiencies in core strength and balance to prevent further injury. The successful integration of history, physical examination, and functional testing will enhance your evaluation of the injured runner and help return athletes to sport.

REFERENCES

1. Kanis JA, Johansson H, Oden A, et al. A meta-analysis of prior corticosteroid use and fracture risk. J Bone Miner Res 2004;19(6):893–9.
2. Hile AM, Anderson JM, Fiala KA, et al. Creatine supplementation and anterior compartment pressure during exercise in the heat in dehydrated men. J Athl Train 2006;41(1):30–5.
3. Kelsey JL, Bachrach LK, Procter-Gray E, et al. Risk factors for stress fracture among young female cross-country runners. Med Sci Sports Exerc 2007;39(9):1457–63.
4. Beck TJ, Ruff CB, Shaffer RA, et al. Stress fracture in military recruits: gender differences in muscle and bone susceptibility factors. Bone 2000;27(3):437–44.
5. Bijur PE, Horodyski M, Egerton W, et al. Comparison of injury during cadet basic training by gender. Arch Pediatr Adolesc Med 1997;151(5):456–61.
6. Korpelainen R, Orava S, Karpakka J, et al. Risk factors for recurrent stress fractures in athletes. Am J Sports Med 2001;29(3):304–10.
7. Plastaras CT, Rittenberg JD, Rittenberg KE, et al. Comprehensive functional evaluation of the injured runner. Phys Med Rehabil Clin North Am 2005;16(3):623–49.
8. Hreljac A. Impact and overuse injuries in runners. Med Sci Sports Exerc 2004;36(5): 845–9.
9. Fredericson M, Rittenberg JD, Rittenberg KE, et al. Tibial stress reaction in runners. Correlation of clinical symptoms and scintigraphy with a new magnetic resonance imaging grading system. Am J Sports Med 1995;23(4):472–81.
10. Boden BP, Osbahr DC. High-risk stress fractures: evaluation and treatment. J Am Acad Orthop Surg 2000;8(6): 344–53.
11. Reider B. The orthopaedic physical examination. Philadelphia: W.B. Saunders; 1999. p. 402.
12. Macdonald SG, Ganz R. Clinical evaluation of the symptomatic young adult hip. Semin Arthroplasty 1997;(8):3–9.
13. Ober FB. The role of the iliotibial and fascia lata as a factor in the causation of low-back disabilities and sciatica. J Bone Joint Surg 1936;18:105.
14. Conley S, Rosenberg A, Crowninshield R. The female knee: anatomic variations. J Am Acad Orthop Surg 2007;15(Suppl 1):S31–6.
15. Messier SP, Davis SE, Curl WW, et al. Etiologic factors associated with patellofemoral pain in runners. Med Sci Sports Exerc 1991;23(9):1008–15.
16. Shultz SJ, Nguyen AD, Windley TC, et al. Intratester and intertester reliability of clinical measures of lower extremity anatomic characteristics: implications for multicenter studies. Clin J Sport Med 2006;16(2):155–61.
17. Brody DM. Techniques in the evaluation and treatment of the injured runner. Orthop Clin North Am 1982;13(3):541–58.
18. Kaufman KR, Brodine SK, Shaffer RA, et al. The effect of foot structure and range of motion on musculoskeletal overuse injuries. Am J Sports Med 1999;27(5):585–93.

19. Crossley KM, Zhang WJ, Schache AG, et al. Performance on the single-leg squat task indicates hip abductor muscle function. Am J Sports Med 2011;39(4):866–73.
20. Willson JD, Ireland ML, Davis I. Core strength and lower extremity alignment during single leg squats. Med Sci Sports Exerc 2006;38(5):945–52.
21. Newton RU, Gerber A, Nimphius S, et al. Determination of functional strength imbalance of the lower extremities. J Strength Cond Res 2006;20(4):971–7.
22. Ryan MB, Valiant GA, McDonald K, et al. The effect of three different levels of footwear stability on pain outcomes in women runners: a randomised control trial. Br J Sports Med 2011;45(9): 715–21.
23. Reynolds G. Are we built to run barefoot? 2011. Available at: http://well.blogs.nytimes.com/2011/06/08/are-we-built-to-run-barefoot/. Accessed July 12, 2011.
24. Jenkins DW, Cauthon DJ. Barefoot running claims and controversies: a review of the literature. J Am Podiatr Med Assoc 2011;101(3):231–46.
25. Divert C, Mornieux G, Baur H, et al. Mechanical comparison of barefoot and shod running. Int J Sports Med 2005;26(7):593–8.
26. Squadrone R, Gallozzi C. Biomechanical and physiological comparison of barefoot and two shod conditions in experienced barefoot runners. J Sports Med Phys Fitness 2009;49(1):6–13.
27. Robbins SE, Hanna AM. Running-related injury prevention through barefoot adaptations. Med Sci Sports Exerc 1987;19(2):148–56.
28. Ogon M, Aleksiev AR, Spratt KF, et al. Footwear affects the behavior of low back muscles when jogging. Int J Sports Med 2001;22(6):414–9.
29. Giuliani J, Masini B, Alitz C, et al. Barefoot-simulating footwear associated with metatarsal stress injury in 2 runners. Orthopedics 2011;34(7):e320–3.
30. Collier R. The rise of barefoot running. CMAJ 2011;183(1):e37–8.

Diagnostic Imaging in the Evaluation of Leg Pain in Athletes

Michael Bresler, MD*, Winnie Mar, MD, Jordan Toman, MD

KEYWORDS

• Radiology • Athletes • Leg pain • Imaging

Acute and chronic leg pain are common clinical problems in both competitive and recreational athletes. Diagnostic considerations include more common injuries, such as medial tibial stress syndrome, stress fracture, Achilles tendon disorders, and hamstring injury as well as less-common conditions, such as chronic exertional compartment syndrome and popliteal artery entrapment syndrome.

History and clinical examination are often sufficient for diagnosis. Diagnostic imaging, however, is essential to differentiate between injuries that may have a common clinical presentation as well as determine the degree of injury. In addition, radiologic evaluation plays a critical role in aiding the clinician in determining underlying causes for some of these conditions, in estimating time required before return to athletic activity, and in documenting healing before return to sport. This article reviews the imaging findings as well as the modalities that are utilized in evaluating both common and uncommon causes of leg pain in athletes.

STRESS INJURY TO BONE

Bone injuries are a major contributor to leg pain in the running athlete. In particular, stress injuries are thought to represent up to approximately 10% of all injuries seen in sports medicine clinics. The majority of these injuries involve the tibia, followed in decreasing frequency by the tarsal bones, metatarsals, femur, and fibula.[1] Imaging plays a major role in the identification of the spectrum of repetitive stress injury to bone, ranging from bone marrow edema to stress fracture. This article reviews the radiographic options, their roles in diagnosis, and their applicability to the most common location of such injuries. Early detection is crucial to prevent stress fracture and its complications.[2]

Tibial stress injuries are the most common cause of lower leg pain in the athlete.[3] They result from abnormal repetitive stress on a normal bone. The resultant bone

The authors have nothing to disclose.
Department of Radiology, University of Illinois at Chicago Medical Center, 1740 West Taylor Street, Room 2483, (M/C 931), Chicago, IL 60612, USA
* Corresponding author.
E-mail address: bresler1@uic.edu

Clin Sports Med 31 (2012) 217–245
doi:10.1016/j.csm.2011.09.006
0278-5919/12/$ – see front matter © 2012 Elsevier Inc. All rights reserved.

injuries vary widely and include such entities as asymptomatic osteopenia, periostitis, cortical fracture, and reactive soft tissue and bone marrow edema.[3–5] Medial tibial stress syndrome (shin splints) usually involves the middle and distal one-third of the tibia and is typically seen in runners. It is thought to be caused by stress reaction of the fascia, periosteum, and bone.[6] It is seen more frequently in women and their risk for progression to stress fracture is much greater (12 times) than their male counterparts.[6]

Radiographs are frequently the first imaging modality used for assessment of lower leg pain. Radiographic manifestations of stress injuries include decreased cortical density, periosteal reaction, endosteal thickening, and a cortical fracture line.[7,8–12] Radiographs are insensitive for the detection of early stress-related injuries[7,13–16] and are only specific if a fracture line is detected.[17] Despite their relative insensitivity, if periosteal reaction is identified on radiographs at the site of the patient's clinical symptoms, it may be assumed that the patient has a high-grade stress injury and should be treated accordingly.[7]

Multiple additional imaging options exist for the patient with lower leg pain. Nuclear scintigraphy, computed tomography (CT) and magnetic resonance imaging (MRI) have all been used for evaluation of these patients with varying degree of success. Nuclear medicine scintigraphy (bone scan) has historically been used to evaluate patients with tibial pain suggestive of stress injury. Bone scan is able to detect subtle changes in bone metabolism well before these changes become evident on conventional radiographs; hence, it can contribute to the early diagnosis.[8] A normal bone scan, however, does not always exclude the presence of a stress reaction.[17] This was shown in a study of 3 military recruits[18] with clinically documented tibial pain, who had originally negative bone scan that became positive 1 month after continued stress. Similarly, CT has been used for assessment, because it is superior to radiographs at detecting subtle periosteal reaction. In a study by Gaeta and colleagues,[2] CT detected more stress-related cortical abnormalities than did MRI. Specifically, CT was better able to detect such cortical findings as osteopenia, resorption cavities, and striations. CT can appear normal in the early stages of stress injury. CT is unable to detect cancellous bone marrow edema or bone bruise, thus, limiting its utility.

Many investigators recommend MRI as the modality of choice for assessment of patients with tibial pain.[2,7,19] Gaeta and colleagues[4] compared the sensitivity and specificity of bone scan, CT, and MRI for detection of stress injuries of the tibia. The sensitivities of MRI, CT, and scintigraphy in the detection of stress injuries was 88%, 42%, and 74%, respectively. The specificity, accuracy, positive predictive value, and negative predictive value were 100%, 90%, 100%, and 62% for MRI and 100%, 52%, 100%, and 26% for CT, respectively.

MR imaging protocols must include a fat-suppressed, fluid-sensitive sequence, such as inversion recovery imaging; T2 fat-suppressed sequence; or proton-density, fat-suppressed sequences. T1-weighted images, which optimize soft tissue contrast, are typically used as well for better depiction of anatomy. On T1-weighted sequences, marrow edema is seen as intermediate or low signal within the otherwise bright marrow. Conversely, marrow or soft tissue edema on fat-suppressed fluid-sensitive sequences is seen as high signal superimposed on the otherwise dark signal of normal marrow. An MRI classification system grading stress-related injuries to the tibia has been developed by Fredericson and colleagues (**Table 1**).[17]

Periostitis or shin splints correspond to a grade 1 stress injury (**Fig. 1**). The earliest indication of medial tibial stress syndrome is hyperintense edema along the medial border of the tibia on fluid-sensitive, fat-suppressed sequences. Soft tissue edema may progress to osseous cortical and marrow changes as outlined

Table 1	
MRI grading of stress injuries to the tibia	
Grade 1	Periosteal edema: mild to moderate on T2-weighted images; Marrow: normal on T1- and T2-weighted images
Grade 2	Periosteal edema: moderate to severe on T2-weighted images; Marrow edema on T2-weighted images
Grade 3	Periosteal edema: moderate to severe on T2-weighted images; Marrow edema on T1- and T2-weighted images
Grade 4	Periosteal edema: moderate to severe on T2-weighted images; Marrow edema on T1- and T2-weighted images, fracture line clearly visible

by the classification system. Grades 2 and 3 represent a spectrum of injury that could lead to a defined fracture line if untreated.[6] Grade 4 indicates presence of a discrete fracture line (**Fig. 2**).

Stress fractures of the hip can also occur in the athlete (**Fig. 3**). Our understanding of the complexities of these injuries and their imaging findings is evolving, and some of the theories about the etiologies of these injuries remain hypothetical. Review of the recent literature sheds light on some of the similarities and differences among the spectrum of disease of the hip that ranges from transient osteoporosis of the hip (TOH) to subchondral fracture (SFFH) to true osteonecrosis of the femoral head (ONFH). Transient osteoporosis of the hip is a self-limited cause of hip pain that usually occurs in pregnant women and middle-aged men. Subchondral fractures of the femoral head are uncommon but thought to represent important and underreported causes of leg pain in the athlete. Subchondral fractures of the femoral head have not only been reported to occur as an insufficiency fracture associated with poor bone quality but also as a fatigue fracture in young military recruits who experienced a rapid increase in physical activity. Therefore, it is expected that similar findings may occur in athletes and otherwise healthy people.[20] Transient osteoporosis of the hip has clinical findings that resemble those of a subchondral fracture.[20] In their study, the imaging findings of SFFH without collapse of the femoral head were similar to those of TOH. Imaging findings included diffuse osteopenia, increased radionuclide uptake, and bone marrow edema in the proximal femur. The bone marrow edema is detected as high signal on T2-weighted, fat-suppressed sequences and low signal on T1-weighted images. The only difference was the existence of a subchondral fracture line on MRI. Findings in their study suggest that TOH and SFFH are subchondral bone injuries of differing severity. Subchondral fracture and bone marrow edema also occur in ONFH; therefore, it is possible for SFFH to be misdiagnosed as ONFH.[20] The main radiographic difference between SFFH and ONFH is subtle. In ONFH, an abnormal signal intensity band, representing the outer margin of the necrotic area, exists outside of the subchondral fracture, and the edema of the femoral head occurs outside of this band. In SFFH, no additional abnormal signal band exists, and the edema extends to the subchondral region.[21]

The relative similarities of TOH, SSFH, and spontaneous osteonecrosis of the knee (SONK) (**Fig. 4**) from a radiographic standpoint have caught the attention of several investigators.[22–27] Yamamoto[26] reported the imaging findings of a patient in whom subchondral fractures of the femoral head and medial femoral condyle developed. Adriaensen and coworkers[22] have recently reported on a patient who presented with TOH and later had SONK. Although SONK is thought to have similar imaging characteristics relative to that of the TOH and SFFH, there is a paucity of reported instances of SONK in the athlete or young patient.

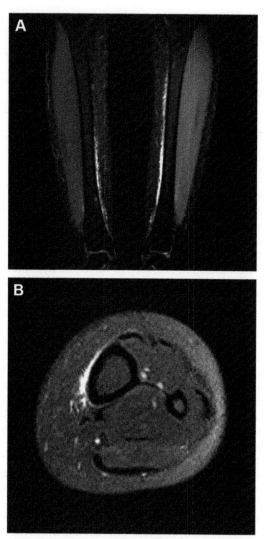

Fig. 1. Thirty-seven-year-old ultramarathon runner with tibial pain and grade 1 injury. Coronal IR image (*A*) and axial T2 fat-suppressed image (*B*) show moderate edema, as evidenced by high signal along the anteromedial cortex.

ACHILLES TENDON INJURIES IN RUNNERS

Runners have a high incidence of Achilles tendon overuse injuries, affecting 11% of runners.[28] These injuries range from paratenonitis to complete tears and are usually caused by overuse of the calf muscles.

The Achilles tendon anteriorly should be generally flat or concave (**Fig. 5**A, B).[29] It can have a small focal convexity anteriorly because of the confluence of the soleus and gastrocnemius muscles, which demonstrate a spiral configuration (see **Fig. 5**C, D).[30] This focal convexity occurs at the lateral aspect of the proximal tendon and medially at its distal aspect.[29] However, the normal tendon should not be diffusely

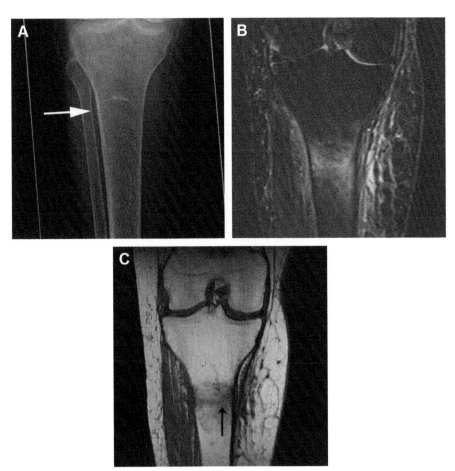

Fig. 2. Patient with chronic intermittent tibial pain. Conventional radiograph (*A*) shows subtle periosteal reaction (*arrow*) along the proximal tibial cortex laterally. T2-weighted, fat-suppressed image (*B*) shows extensive marrow and deep soft tissue edema (high signal). T1-weighted image (*C*) shows edema and subtle fracture line *(black arrow)*.

convex anteriorly. Small, vertically oriented, higher signal structures in the tendon may be normal and represent the confluence of the soleus and gastrocnemius[31] or the confluence of interfascicular membranes nearer the insertion[32] or small vessels. The plantaris tendon is present in 90% of people and is a small tendon located medial to the Achilles tendon (see **Fig. 5**C, D). It should not be mistaken for an Achilles tendon tear.[29]

The Achilles tendon does not have a tendon sheath but rather a paratenon that surrounds it medially, laterally, and posteriorly.[29,30] Paratenonitis (also referred to as *peritendinitis* or *paratendinitis*) is secondary to inflammation and increased fluid of the paratenon (**Fig. 6**).[32,33] The paratenon can also develop fibrous adhesions from chronic inflammation.

On the contrary, degeneration of the tendon is usually referred to as *tendinosis* rather than *tendinitis* because there is no inflammatory cell infiltrate, as is seen with paratenonitis. This usually occurs in a relatively hypovascular zone, which is located

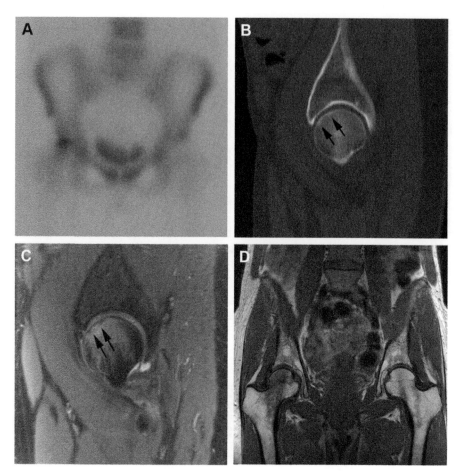

Fig. 3. Forty-seven-year-old runner with progressive right hip pain. Bone scan (*A*) shows abnormal subchondral activity in the right hip. Reformatted sagittal CT (*B*) shows subtle subchondral sclerosis (*arrows*). Proton-density, fat-suppressed sagittal image (*C*) shows subchondral fracture line (*arrows*) with edema extending to the articular surface and into the femoral neck. T1-weighted coronal image of the hips bilaterally (*D*) redemonstrates the extensive edema in the right hip as shown by the lower-signal-intensity marrow relative to the normal contralateral hip.

2 to 6 cm from the tendon insertion.[34,35] Tendinosis can predispose to tears, including spontaneous tendon tears.[36] The most common type of tendon degeneration is termed *hypoxic tendinosis*.[37] It is thought to have an ischemic component secondary to its location in the watershed area of the tendon. In hypoxic tendinosis, the tendon is thickened but retains its hypointense dark signal (**Fig. 7**).

Mucoid degeneration is the second most common form and is usually painless.[32] In mucoid degeneration, there is increased, usually intermediate, ill-defined signal within the thickened tendon. Hypoxic and mucoid degeneration often coexist.[36] Mucoid degeneration may also be confused with interstitial tears.[38] However, interstitial tears occur parallel to the long axis of the tendon.

Insertional tendinitis is associated with an inflammatory cell infiltrate.[33] It is commonly seen in runners[32,39]; per one investigator it is seen in 6.5% to 18% of

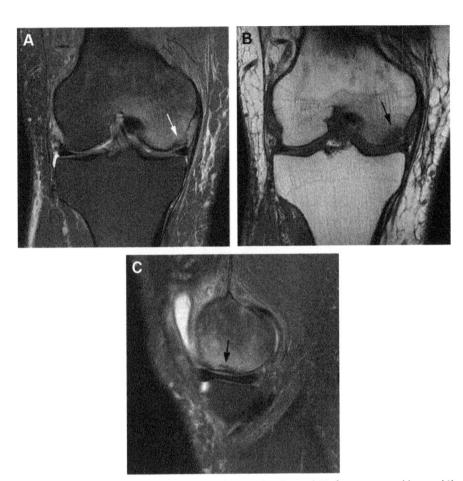

Fig. 4. Middle-aged male with progressive knee pain. Coronal PD fat-suppressed image (*A*) and coronal T1-weighted image (*B*) show subchondral fracture line (*white arrow*) with associated high-signal and low-signal-intensity edema, respectively. Sagittal T2-weighted image (*C*) shows the subchondral fracture, contour deformity of the femoral condyle, and extensive subjacent edema.

runners.[28] It appears as distal tendon thickening with ill-defined longitudinal high signal intensity, which may mimic a partial tear **(Fig. 8)**.[32] This may be associated with Achilles tendon enthesopathy[33]; however, the presence of an enthesophyte does not necessarily imply Achilles tendon disorders.[28]

Retrocalcaneal bursitis is often seen with Achilles tendon disorders, although it can also be present with rheumatologic disorders or as an isolated disorder.[40] It is seen more commonly in the presence of a prominent posterior calcaneal tuberosity known as Haglund's deformity, which is associated with high heel footwear or hockey players with a rigid heel counter. Retrocalcaneal bursitis can also occur in runners without predisposing calcaneal morphology, particularly in uphill runners.[33] Haglund's deformity is often associated with retrocalcaneal bursitis, retro-Achilles bursitis, and insertional tendinitis **(Fig. 9)**.[32,33] The retro-Achilles bursa is posterior to

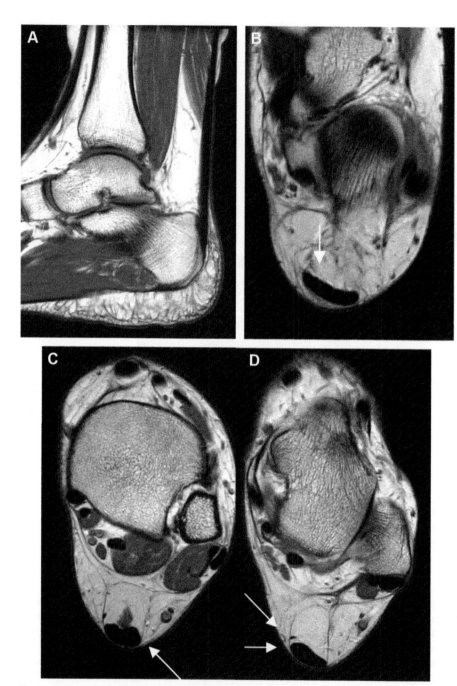

Fig. 5. Sagittal T1 (*A*) shows a normal-sized Achilles tendon without convexity anteriorly. Axial proton density images (*B,C,D*) show the normal flat Achilles tendon (*B*) with parallel anterior and posterior margins. The anterior margin is normally concave (*arrow* in *B*), and the posterior margin is normally convex. Normal slight convexity of the proximal Achilles tendon laterally (*arrow* in *C*), and slight convexity medially more distally (*short arrow* in *D*) is shown. The normal plantaris tendon is indicated by the long arrow (*D*).

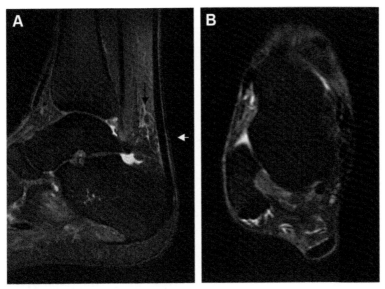

Fig. 6. Sagittal (*A*) and axial (*B*) fat-saturated PD show fluid surrounding the Achilles tendon consistent with paratenonitis (*white arrow*). Edema is also present in Kager's fat pad (*black arrow*). Achilles tendon is normal in size and signal intensity.

the Achilles tendon. The fat posterior to the tendon should always be preserved; if it is not, then this is consistent with retro-Achilles bursitis.[32]

MRI and ultrasound can be useful in differentiating partial from complete Achilles tendon ruptures, as physical examination findings can be obscured by hematoma.[41–43] In a partial tear, there is fluid signal intensity within the tendon, with

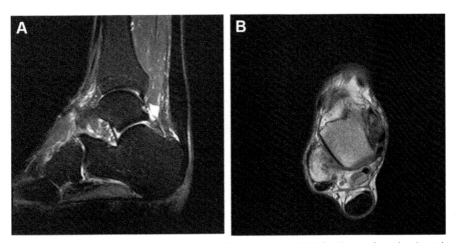

Fig. 7. Sagittal (*A*) and axial fat-saturated PD (*B*) show marked thickening and predominantly hypointense signal of the Achilles tendon centered at the hypovascular zone consistent with tendinosis, hypoxic type.

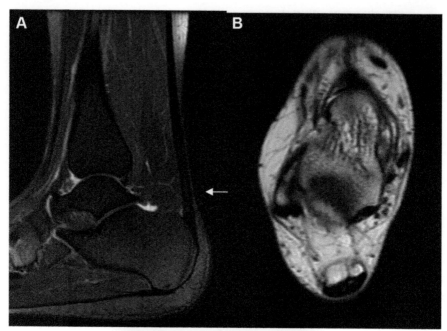

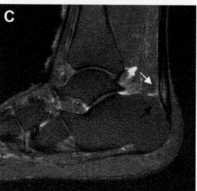

Fig. 8. Sagittal fat saturated PD (*A*) and axial PD (*B*) show increased, intermediate signal intensity in the distal Achilles tendon near the insertion (*arrow*) consistent with insertional tendinitis. Sagittal fat saturated PD image (*C*) shows distal Achilles tendon thickening and longitudinal increased intermediate signal intensity consistent with insertional Achilles tendinitis and an interstitial tendon tear. Note reactive bone marrow edema at the calcaneal attachment (*black arrow*) and mild retrocalcaneal bursitis (*white arrow*).

incomplete extension, more often reaching the posterior surface than the anterior surface.[28] A partial tear can be difficult to distinguish from tendinosis, particularly mucoid degeneration, but ancillary findings, such as surrounding edema/hemorrhage or edema in Kager's fat pad, can help point toward a tear.

A complete tear shows complete fiber disruption with a gap between the torn and retracted tendon edges (**Fig. 10**). It is important to note the size of the gap, the presence of underlying tendinosis of the torn tendon, and muscle atrophy if present. If conservative

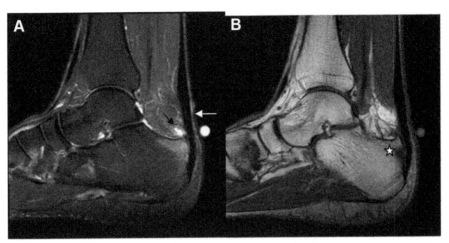

Fig. 9. Sagittal PD fat-saturated (*A*) and sagittal T1 images (*B*) show a prominent posterior calcaneal tuberosity with reactive marrow edema (*star*), insertional Achilles tendinitis, retrocalcaneal (*black arrow*) and pre-Achilles bursitis (*white arrow*), suggestive of Haglund's disease.

treatment is undertaken, imaging can be used to determine if the tendon edges are closely apposed while in the slightly plantarflexed position in the cast.

Tears usually occur in the watershed zone 2 to 6 cm from the insertion. Atypical Achilles tendon tears can occur proximally and distally. A proximal tear is a myotendinous junction injury of the gastrocnemius muscle and is more commonly seen in squash, tennis, or football players rather than runners.[32] Occasionally, the tendon can tear distally at the calcaneal attachment.

Some investigators have stated that there is overlap between the MRI appearance of the Achilles tendon and pain.[30,38,44] Another study found that the presence of calcaneal edema always indicated pain in their series.[38] Haims and coworkers[38] also found that pain was present in all of the patients with complete or partial tears and the majority of interstitial tears and more in hypoxic rather than mucoid degeneration tendinosis.[38] On the contrary, a study by Gärdin and colleagues[44] found that pain was related more to intratendinous signal abnormality rather than tendon enlargement. Trace areas of increased signal intensity within the tendon were commonly found in asymptomatic individuals and were postulated to be a result of small vessels or normal fascial anatomy.[30]

INJURY TO THE HAMSTRING MUSCLE COMPLEX

The hamstring muscle complex is the most frequently injured muscle group in athletes[45] and is not uncommon in runners. More than 50% of muscle strains in sprinters involve the hamstrings.[46] Injury can also occur during stretching.[47] Though hamstring muscle injuries can often be diagnosed clinically, imaging has an important role in differentiating patients needing surgical versus conservative management, optimizing rehabilitation time, and in differentiating hamstring injury from other causes of posterior thigh pain, such as bursitis or referred neurologic pain.[45]

The hamstring muscle complex is made up of 3 muscles: the biceps femoris, semitendinosus, and semimembranosus. The biceps femoris and semitendinosus originate from a common conjoint tendon at the ischial tuberosity. The semimembranosus

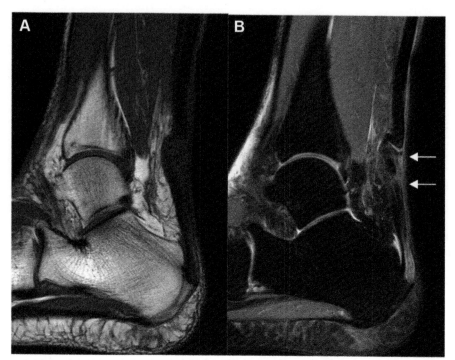

Fig. 10. Sagittal T1 (*A*) and fat-saturated PD (*B*) show a full-thickness Achilles tendon tear at the hypovascular zone. A small gap is present (*arrows*).

muscle has its own origin, also at the ischial tuberosity, but superolateral to the conjoint tendon (**Fig. 11**). Distally, the biceps femoris inserts onto the head of the fibula and lateral tibial condyle, whereas the semitendinosus inserts, along with the gracilis and sartorius muscles, onto the proximal medial tibia, forming the pes anserinus. The semimembranosus courses anterior to the other hamstring muscles and has multiple insertions, including the posteromedial tibial condyle and posteromedial joint capsule. The short head of the biceps muscle originates from the linea aspera and inserts onto the fibular head as well. A portion of the adductor magnus muscle "hamstring head" also originates from the ischial tuberosity and also functions to extend the hip. The sciatic nerve is in close proximity to the proximal hamstring tendon origins and can be affected by hamstring injuries,[48] probably secondary to surrounding hematoma or edema.

The biceps femoris is the most commonly injured hamstring muscle, with several studies debating the frequency of semimembranosus and semitendinosus injury as the least commonly injured muscle.[49] Within any muscle, the myotendinous junction is the most common site of injury.[50,51] The myotendinous junction is defined as an approximately 10- to 12-cm zone in which myofibrils transition into the tendon. The proximal junction, where there is a higher percentage of myofibrils, is more commonly torn than the distal aspect. On fluid-sensitive MR images, fluid and hemorrhage tracking along the torn myofibrils produce the characteristic feathery appearance of hamstring strain. Hamstring tendinosis will show enlargement and increased intermediate signal, but not fluid signal, and

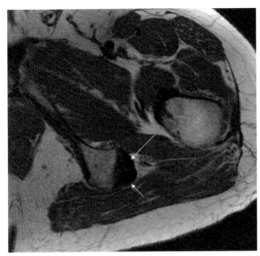

Fig. 11. Axial T1 image at the level of the ischial tuberosity shows hamstring anatomy. Longer white arrow indicates the semimembranosus tendon. Shorter white arrow indicates the conjoint tendon, which consists of the semitendinosus and biceps femoris tendons.

heterogeneity of the tendon. A partial-thickness tear will show a linear, fluid-filled cleft within the tendon (**Figs. 12** and **13**).[47]

In avulsion injuries, the conjoint tendon is the most commonly involved region, with bony avulsion being uncommon. The exception is pediatric patients, in whom bony avulsion is more common secondary to the weakness of the apophysis relative to the tendons. Distal avulsions of the hamstring muscle insertions do occur, but are rare, and are usually seen in patients with chronic hamstring injury as a predisposing factor.[45] Full-thickness hamstring tears or avulsions will show a large, fluid-filled gap between the tendon and ischial tuberosity and possibly tendon retraction (**Fig. 14**). Subacute or chronic ischial avulsions may show mixed lysis and sclerosis and should not be confused with a neoplastic process (**Fig. 15**).[52]

With its exquisite soft tissue contrast and resolution, and lack of ionizing radiation, MRI is the most sensitive imaging study and is the modality of choice for evaluating the hamstring muscle complex.[53] Because increased water content, such as edema, is a hallmark of musculoskeletal injuries, fluid-sensitive sequences such as T2 and short tau inversion recovery (STIR) are usually the most helpful.[54] A T1 sequence should also be included for improved anatomic delineation and for the detection of hemorrhage or fatty muscle atrophy. In addition to detecting the presence of hamstring injury, several studies examining professional athletes have found that the total area of muscle involved on MRI strongly correlates with the length of rehabilitation and time to return to athletic activity.[55]

Ultrasonography is also a sensitive imaging modality for evaluating injury to the hamstring muscle complex, demonstrating fluid collections around injured muscle as well as increased echogenicity in muscles containing edema and hemorrhage. A study of 60 professional athletes, in whom both ultrasound scan and MRI were performed in the acute phase of injury as well as at 2 and 6 weeks postinjury, showed that both MRI and ultrasound scan were accurate in detecting hamstring injury in the acute phase (0–3 days). The few cases in which acute injury was detected by MRI but not ultrasound scan were very mild strains in which there was minimal edema but no hemorrhage or disruption

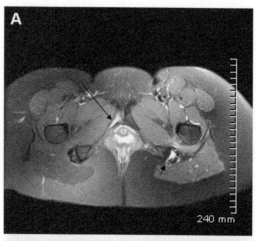

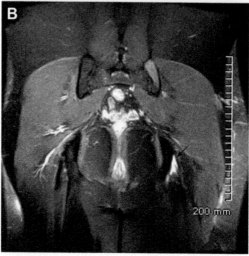

Fig. 12. Axial (*A*) and coronal (*B*) fluid-sensitive sequences show a fluid-filled cleft (*short arrow* in *A* and *B*) at the left conjoint tendon, with some intact fibers remaining, and no muscle retraction. This is compatible with a partial tear. Stress reaction in the anterior right pubic body was also present (*long arrow*). (*Courtesy of* Amir Sepahdari, MD.)

of muscle architecture. At both 2 and 6 weeks postinjury, MRI was shown to be more sensitive than ultrasound scan.[51] However, ultrasound scan can be very sensitive in the detection of injuries to the distal hamstring tendons because of the superficial location of these injuries.

EXERTIONAL COMPARTMENT SYNDROME

Chronic exertional compartment syndrome results from increased compartment pressures in a limited fibro-osseous compartment. This most commonly occurs in the lower leg and the volar forearm. In the lower leg, the anterior compartment is most commonly affected, and symptoms often occur during strenuous exercise, such as running. Noncompliant fascia, on top of increased muscle bulk and muscle microtears, contribute to increased pressures.[56]

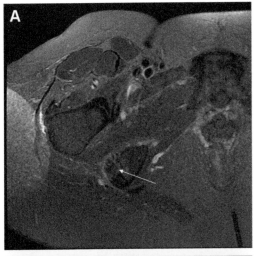

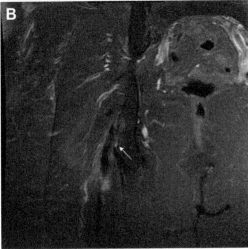

Fig. 13. Axial (*A*) and coronal (*B*) proton density, fat-saturated images show intermediate signal and thickening of the semimembranosus tendon (*arrow* in *A*) consistent with tendinosis, along with a small partial tear and reactive bone marrow edema of the ischial tuberosity (*arrow* in *B*).

Increased muscle interstitial edema results in increased pressure in the compartment but usually leaves no permanent damage on the muscles.[57] This increased pressure can compromise blood flow to the compartment and result in temporary muscle and nerve ischemia. Pain is always present and typically described as cramping, aching, tightness, or burning. Neurologic symptoms may also be present.

The gold standard is direct measurement of compartment pressures. Imaging can be performed as an ancillary study or in special circumstances when the patient refuses pressure measurements or has a contraindication, such as anticoagulation.[58] MRI is the imaging modality of choice. It has been shown to have statistically significant T2 signal increases in this syndrome.[59–61] Some also showed that these findings resolved after

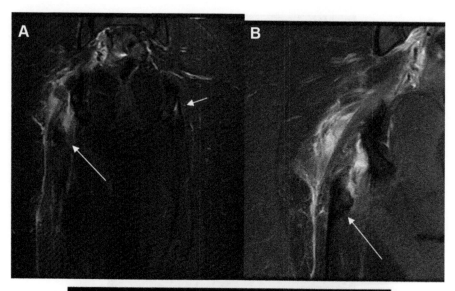

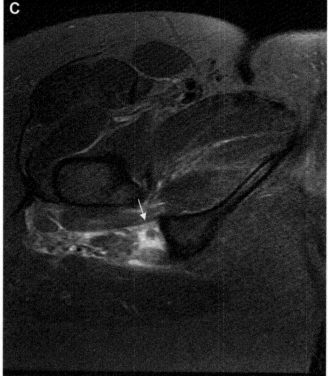

Fig. 14. (*A*) Large field of view (FOV) coronal STIR (*A*), small FOV coronal (*B*), and axial (*C*) fat-saturated PD images show the full-thickness right hamstring tendon tear with a large fluid-filled gap (*short arrow* in *C*) and retraction of the hamstring tendons (*long arrows*). Large FOV coronal STIR also shows a partial tear of the contralateral left hamstring tendons (*short arrow* in *A*).

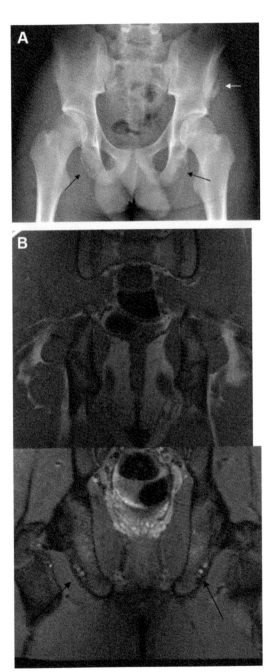

Fig. 15. Frontal view of the hip (*A*) shows cystic changes of both ischial tuberosities secondary to chronic avulsive hamstring stress (*black arrows*). The patient also has a sartorius avulsion of the left anterior superior iliac crest (*white arrows*). (*B*) Coronal T1 (*above*) and coronal STIR (*below*) show chronic avulsive stress to the bilateral ischial tuberosity apophyses with cystic changes (*arrows*).

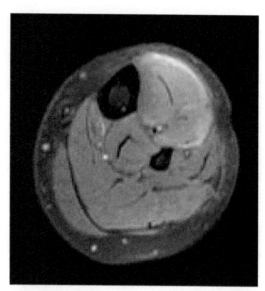

Fig. 16. Postexercise T2-weighted, fat-saturated image shows increased T2 signal intensity edema in the anterior compartment, secondary to exertional anterior compartment syndrome. Pre-exercise images were normal. (*Courtesy of* Andrew Sonin, MD.)

fasciotomy.[59,61] MRI has the advantage of also showing other findings, which may cause pain, such as medial tibial stress syndrome.[58]

The hallmark of this pathology is increased T2 signal intensity, which is thought to correspond to interstitial muscle edema, typically shortly after exercise, that may persist up to 25 minutes after the exercise is completed.

Imaging must be performed both before and after exercise, because rest images are usually normal. An adequate delay to show resolution of edema is also necessary. The patient should perform enough exercise to reproduce symptoms. Exercise may be performed by running. Imaging should be performed within 1 minute of the completion of exercise, however. To lessen delay between exercise and scan time, repeated dorsiflexion and plantar flexion against resistance while in the scanner has also been used,[62–64] and was enough to reproduce symptoms and show imaging findings.

The MRI protocol should consist of mainly fluid-sensitive sequences, such as STIR, T2, or proton density (PD). Fat saturation will increase conspicuity of edema. At least one T1-weighted image should also be included for better anatomic detail. The axial plane is the most important. The main finding is increased T2 signal intensity on postexercise images. Compartmental bulging, convex deep fascial margins, and effacement of the fascial planes may also be seen (**Fig. 16**).[56]

Because the legs are commonly bilaterally involved,[56,65] imaging of both legs in the same field of view can be helpful. Multiple and asymmetric muscle groups may also be involved[65] and may not be measured or easily measurable, such as the deep posterior compartment. Contrast does not have to be used, but there are reports that it may increase the sensitivity for postexercise findings in the form of increased enhancement of the affected muscles (**Fig. 17**).

Muscle herniations through fascial defects can be identified in up to 40% of cases of suspected exertional compartment syndrome.[56] This entity itself can also cause pain in runners. A focal bulge of muscle, and sometimes a fascial defect, will be seen. This often

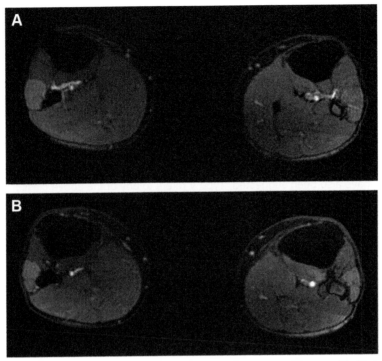

Fig. 17. Postexercise, postcontrast T1 gradient echo fat-saturated images (*A, B*) show increased enhancement and bulging of the right peroneus longus and brevis muscles, secondary to exertional lateral compartment syndrome. Pre-exercise images were normal.

correlates to an area in which the patient feels a bulge or hard mass. Dorsiflexed, plantarflexed, or dynamic cine images may accentuate these herniations.[66]

As described above, several studies have found that a statistically significant increased T2 muscle signal can be seen postexercise. One group found a statistically increased T1 signal in those with compartment pressure greater than 40 mm Hg after exercise[60] but no significant increase in T2 signal; subsequent studies have not used T1 as their primary measurement in chronic exertional compartment syndrome. Varying results in different studies could be related to different cutoffs of pressure measurements for their symptomatic group, making comparison between studies difficult. The degree of MRI findings has been linked to the degree of compartment pressure,[60] and the lower cutoff used by some groups may have skewed their data. The timing between end of exercise and imaging also varied. One group has devised a special coil so that imaging can be performed during isometric exercises and without any significant delay postexercise.[64] Other novel methods to detect changes, such as increased deoxygenated hemoglobin and restricted water motion, have not shown a statistically significant difference between symptomatic subjects and controls.[63,67] Near-infrared spectroscopy measuring tissue venous oxygen saturation has been shown to correlate well with exertional compartment syndrome.[61] Further work is needed to determine the role of imaging in this syndrome.

POPLITEAL ARTERY ENTRAPMENT SYNDROME

Popliteal artery entrapment syndrome (PAES) is a rare entity, with a reported incidence of 0.165 to 3.5%.[68] It occurs predominantly in men, and patients are typically under the age of 50 and athletic. Patients present with symptoms of lower extremity claudication or rest pain.

Popliteal artery entrapment occurs in patients with abnormal embryologic development of a muscle or tendon or abnormal course of the popliteal artery within the popliteal fossa. Four types of PAES have been described and classified according to Whelen-Rich.[68–70] Type I occurs when the popliteal artery courses medial to the medial head of the gastrocnemius, rather than its normal course between the medial and lateral heads of this muscle. In type II, the arterial course is normal, but the medial head of the gastrocnemius arises from an abnormal lateral position. In type III, an abnormal slip of muscle arises from the gastrocnemius and compresses the popliteal artery. Type IV occurs when an abnormal fibrous band, or when the popliteus muscle, compresses the popliteal artery. Two additional types, not originally described by Whelan, have also been suggested. Type V refers to any of the above classifications that also involve the popliteal vein. Type VI occurs when the popliteal fossa anatomy is normal, but hypertrophy of the surrounding musculature compresses the popliteal artery (functional PAES) (**Fig. 18**).[71–73]

Several imaging modalities can be used to confirm the diagnosis of popliteal artery entrapment. Traditionally, angiography has been considered the imaging modality of choice because of its ability to diagnose arterial pathologies associated with PAES, including occlusive or partially occlusive thrombosis, ectasia, or aneurysm. In noncomplicated PAES, the typical findings seen with angiography are a normal popliteal artery lumen in neutral position and narrowing of the arterial lumen with stress angiography (performed with patient in active plantar flexion). Conventional angiography can also show abnormal course of the popliteal artery (type I PAES). Less-desirable features inherent in using conventional angiography for the diagnosis of PAES include inability to delineate other anatomic causes of entrapment, such as abnormal muscle or tendon slips, and inability to differentiate entrapment from other causes of popliteal artery disease, such as atherosclerosis. Additionally, angiography is an invasive procedure requiring radiation, conscious sedation, and iodinated contrast administration.[71,72]

Cross-sectional techniques, such as MRI, have the ability to delineate the abnormal relationship between the popliteal artery and surrounding musculotendinous structures. MRI is preferable because of the lack of ionizing radiation and the ability to obtain real-time angiographic images, which allows imaging in dorsiflexion, flexion, and neutral positions. When more complex flow dynamics are involved, such as when there is stenosis or aneurysm of the artery, gadolinium contrast-enhanced MRI can be considered to better delineate the popliteal artery lumen (**Figs. 19 and 20**).[74] MR angiography has been shown in several studies to adequately detect popliteal artery compression when scanning is performed in neutral position and active plantar flexion.[71,74]

Imaging evaluation of both lower extremities should be performed both with standard MRI sequences and MR angiography, even in patients with unilateral symptoms, because bilateral involvement is seen in 30% to 60% of patients.[68] Although MRI of both lower extremities can be performed simultaneously using a torso or head coil, image quality is significantly improved when imaging is performed separately using extremity coils. Computed tomography angiography (CTA) may be advantageous for this purpose, because both extremities may be scanned simultaneously, with a single-contrast bolus, while maintaining good image resolution. Although the delineation of soft tissue anatomy by CT is less optimal than MR, CTA more accurately shows the extravascular anatomy when compared with conventional angiography. In addition, CTA takes less time to complete than MRI, and may

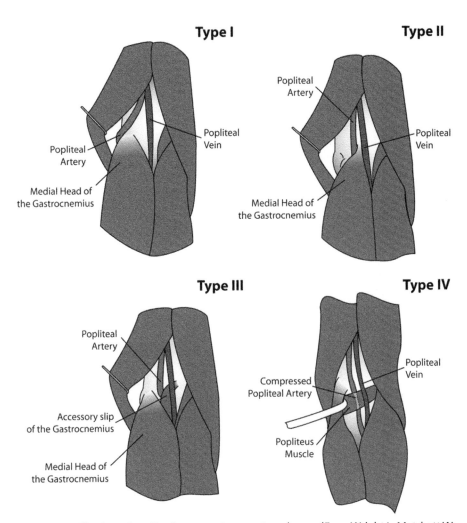

Fig. 18. Classification of popliteal artery entrapment syndrome. (*From* Wright L, Matchett W, Cruz C, et al. Popliteal artery disease: diagnosis and treatment. Radiographics 2004;24:467–79; with permission.)

produce better image quality in patients who are unable to hold a plantar flexed position for the duration of MRI scanning, or who may have other contraindications to MRI.[68]

Imaging findings diagnostic of PAES are similar in both MRI and CT. Both modalities are sensitive at showing popliteal artery narrowing with stress imaging, and both can accurately delineate abnormal anatomic relationships in the popliteal fossa, including abnormal course of the popliteal artery and presence of anomalous tendon or muscle slips causing extrinsic arterial compression.[68] In addition, cross-sectional imaging is also superior in its ability to differentiate PAES from other causes of popliteal artery disease, including popliteal artery aneurysm, cystic adventitial disease, atherosclerotic disease, and arterial compression by other abnormal structures (eg, compression by an adjacent osteochondroma) (**Fig. 21**).

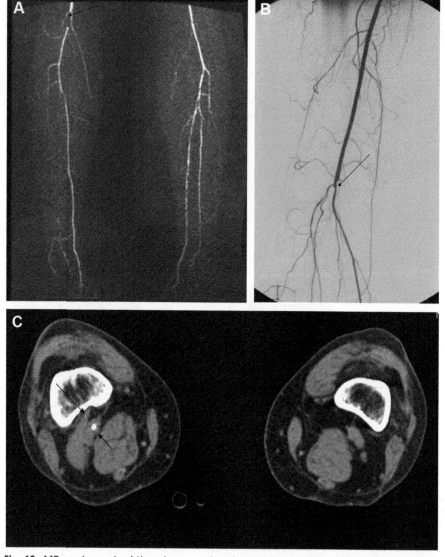

Fig. 19. MR angiography (*A*) and conventional angiography (*B*), performed in the same patient during active plantar flexion, show flow limiting stenosis (*arrow* in *A*) and complete occlusion (*arrow* in *B*) of the right popliteal artery. Axial noncontrast CT images of both lower extremities show abnormal lateral insertion of the medial head of the gastrocnemius on the right (*long arrow* in *C*), and normal popliteal fossa anatomy on the left. Angiography catheter is present in the right popliteal artery (*short arrow* in *C*). (*Courtesy of* Ron Gaba, MD.)

Cystic adventitial disease (CAD) is a rare condition that presents similar to PAES, with symptoms of claudication, typically in young males. CAD causes arterial compression as a result of mucoid cysts, which develop in the adventitial layer of the vessel, and can grow large. Despite its rare occurrence, 85% of CAD

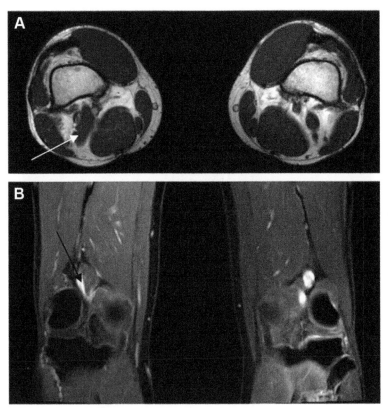

Fig. 20. Ax T1 (*A*) of bilateral knees in a different patient shows an anomalous head of the medial gastrocnemius interposed between the popliteal artery and vein on the right (*arrow*). Note the normal lack of muscle between the artery and vein in the left knee. Postcontrast coronal T1 gradient echo fat-saturated images (*B*) show narrowing of the right popliteal artery in the region of the anomalous muscle (*arrow*). Normal appearance of the left popliteal fossa is shown for comparison.

occurs in the popliteal artery.[73] Conventional angiography will only show narrowing of the artery, but T2-weighted images of the popliteal fossa will demonstrate hyperintense cysts expanding the adventitial layer and compressing the arterial lumen (**Fig. 22**).

SUMMARY

The causes of leg pain in the athlete are diverse. Pain can relate to more common etiologies, such as musculotendinous injury to the hamstrings and Achilles tendon as well as stress injury to bone, with tibial stress injuries comprising the most common cause for lower leg pain in athletes. Less-common causes include chronic exertional compartment syndrome and popliteal artery entrapment syndrome, both of which cause pain as a result of muscle ischemia.

Radiologic evaluation plays an important role in differentiating among the many possible causes of leg pain and is often essential in determining degree of injury as well as in documenting healing before patient return to athletic activity. With

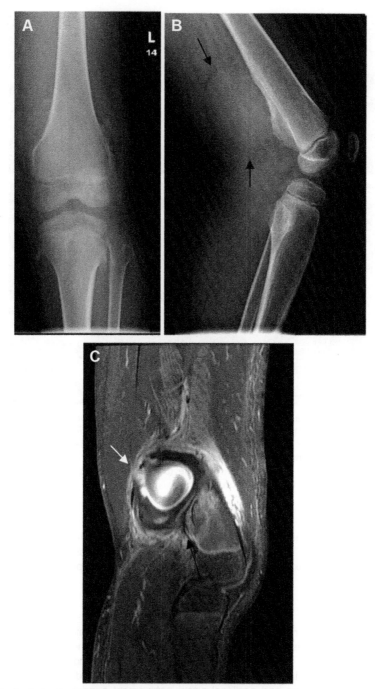

Fig. 21. Frontal (*A*) and lateral (*B*) radiographs show multiple hereditary exostoses and a large soft tissue density rounded mass in the popliteal fossa (*arrows*). Sagittal T1 fat-saturated postcontrast MR image (*C*) of the left knee shows a large pseudoaneurysm of the popliteal artery abutting the posterior distal femur sessile osteochondroma (*black arrow*). The popliteal artery connection to the aneurysm is shown with a white arrow.

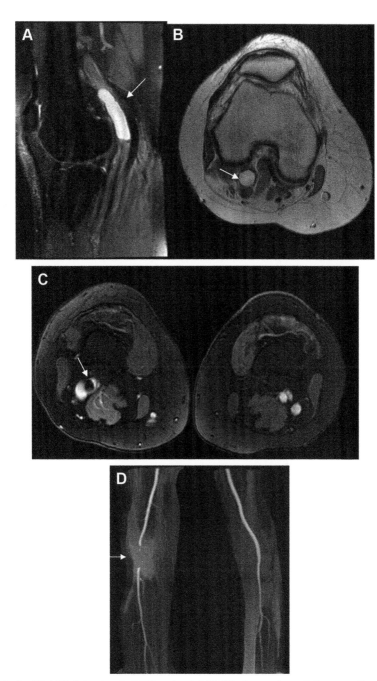

Fig. 22. Sagittal PD fat-saturated (A) and axial PD (B) show a hyperintense cystic structure adjacent to the popliteal artery resulting in significant mass effect on it (*white arrow*). The adjacent popliteal vein is posterior. (C) Postcontrast axial T1 gradient echo fat-saturated images show extrinsic narrowing of the popliteal artery by this T1 hypointense, nonenhancing cyst (*white arrow*). (D) Maximum intensity projection images from an MRA show narrowing of the popliteal artery (*white arrow*), the cause of which is seen on the preceding nonangiographic images.

PAES and hamstring and Achilles injuries, imaging may be helpful in surgical planning as well as in determining an underlying anatomic cause for injury. Several of these conditions can be evaluated with multiple different imaging modalities. The imaging modality of choice should be selected based on the sensitivity and specificity of the imaging examination but should also be tailored to each individual patient after determining comorbidities that may preclude certain types of imaging as well as assessing the patient's ability to undergo such testing.

REFERENCES

1. Matheson GO, Clement DB, McKenzie DC, et al. Stress fractures in athletes: a study of 320 cases. Am J Sports Med 1987;15:46–58.
2. Gaeta M, Minutolli F, Scribano E, et al. CT and MR imaging findings in athletes with early tibial stress injuries: comparison with bone scintigraphy findings and emphasis on cortical abnormalities. Radiology 2005;235:553–61.
3. Anderson MW, Greenspan A. Stress fractures. Radiology 1996;199:1–12.
4. Gaeta M, Minutoli F, Scribano E, et al. CT and MRI findings in athletes with early tibial stress injuries: comparison with bone scintigraphy and emphasis on cortical abnormalities. Radiology 2005;235:553–61.
5. Gaeta M, Minutoli F, Vinci S, et al. High-resolution CT grading of tibial stress reactions in distance runners. AJR 2006;187:789–93.
6. Stoller D. Magnetic resonance imaging in orthopaedics and sports medicine. Baltimore (MD) and Philadelphia (PA): Lippincott Williams and Wilkins; 2007.
7. Kijowski R, Choi J, Mukharjee, et al. Significance of radiographic abnormalities in patients with tibial stress injuries: correlation with magnetic resonance imaging. Skeletal Radiol 2007;36:633–40.
8. Anderson MW, Greenspan A. Stress fractures. Radiology 1996;199:1–12.
9. Daffner RH, Martinez S, Gehweiler JA Jr, et al. Stress fractures of the proximal tibia in runners. Radiology 1982;142:63–5.
10. Mulligan ME. The "gray cortex": an early sign of stress fracture. Skeletal Radiol 1995;24:201–3.
11. Sofka CM. Imaging of stress fractures. Clin Sports Med 2006;25:53–62.
12. Gaeta M, Minutoli F, Mazziotti S, et al. Diagnostic imaging in athletes with chronic lower leg pain. AJR 2008;141219.
13. Giladi M, Nili E, Ziv Y, et al. Comparison between radiography, bone scan, and ultrasound in the diagnosis of stress fractures. Mil Med 1984;149:459–61.
14. Greaney RB, Gerber FH, Laughlin RL, et al. Distribution and natural history of stress fractures in U.S. Marine recruits. Radiology 1983;146:339–46.
15. Prather JL, Nusynowitz ML, Snowdy HA, et al. Scintigraphic findings in stress fractures. J Bone Joint Surg Am 1977;59:869–74.
16. Zwas ST, Elkanovitch R, Frank G. Interpretation and classification of bone scintigraphic findings in stress fractures. J Nucl Med 1987;28:452–7.
17. Fredericson M, Bergman G, Hoffman K, et al. Tibial stress reaction in runners correlation of clinical symptoms and scintigraphy with a new magnetic resonance imaging grading system. Am J Sports Med 1995;23:472–81.
18. Milgrom C, Chisin R, Giladi M, et al. Negative bone scans in impending tibial stress fractures. A report of 3 cases. Am J Sports Med 1985;13:87–94.
19. Harrast M, Colonno D. Stress fractures in runners. Clin Sports Med 2009;29:399–416.
20. Kim JW, Yoo JJ, Min BW, et al. Subchondral fracture of the femoral head in healthy adults. Clin Orthop Relat Res 2007;464:196–204.

21. Song WS, Yoo JJ, Koo KH, et al. Subchondral fatigue fracture of the femoral head in military recruits. Bone Joint Surg Am 2004; 86–A(9):1917–24.

22. Adriaensen ME, Mulhall KJ, Borghans RA, et al. Transient osteoporosis of the hip and spontaneous osteonecrosis of the knee: a common aetiology? Ir J Med Sci 2009. [Epub ahead of print].

23. Miyanishi K, Kaminomachi S, Hara T, et al. A subchondral fracture in transient osteoporosis of the hip. Skeletal Radiol 2007;36(7):677–80.

24. Ramnath RR, Kattapuram SV. MR appearance of SONK-like subchondral abnormalities in the adult knee: SONK redefined. Skeletal Radiol 2004;33(10):575–81.

25. Sokoloff RM, Farooki S, Resnick D. Spontaneous osteonecrosis of the knee associated with ipsilateral tibial plateau stress fracture: report of two patients and review of the literature. Skeletal Radiol 2001:30(1):53–6.

26. Yamamoto T, Bullough PG. Subchondral insufficiency fracture of the femoral head and medial femoral condyle. Skeletal Radiol 2000;29(1):40–4.

27. Miyanishi K, Yamamoto T, Nakashima Y, et al. Subchondral changes in transient osteoporosis of the hip. Skeletal Radiol 2001;30(5):255–61.

28. Stoller D. The ankle and foot. In: Magnetic resonance imaging in orthopaedics and sports medicine. Baltimore (MD) and Philadelphia (PA): Lippincott Williams and Wilkins; 2007. p. 826–49.

29. Kaplan P. Musculoskeletal MRI. Philadelphia (PA): WB Saunders Company; 2001. p. 395–7.

30. Soila K, Karjalainen PT, Aronen HJ, et al. High-resolution MR imaging of the asymptomatic Achilles tendon: new observations. AJR 1999;173(2):323–8.

31. Kong A, Cassumbhoy R, Subramaniam RM. Magnetic resonance imaging of ankle tendons and ligaments: part I–anatomy. Australas Radiol 2007;51(4):315–23.

32. Schweitzer ME, Karasick D. MR imaging of disorders of the Achilles tendon. AJR 2000;175:613–25.

33. Schepsis AA, Jones H, Haas AL. Achilles tendon disorders in athletes. Am J Sports Med 2002;30(2):287–305.

34. Clement DB, Taunton JE, Smart GW. Achilles tendinitis and peritendinitis: etiology and treatment. Am J Sports Med 1984;12(3):179–84.

35. Lagergren C, Lindholm A. Vascular distribution in the Achilles tendon: an angiographic and microangiographic study. Acta Chir Scand 1959;116(5-6):491–5.

36. Kannus P, Józsa L. Histopathological changes preceding spontaneous rupture of a tendon. A controlled study of 891 patients. J Bone Joint Surg Am 1991;73(10): 1507–25.

37. Fox JM, Blazina ME, Jobe FW, et al. Degeneration and rupture of the Achilles tendon. Clin Orthop Relat Res 1975;(107): 221–4.

38. Haims AH, Schweitzer ME, Patel RS, et al. MR imaging of the Achilles tendon: overlap of findings in symptomatic and asymptomatic individuals. Skeletal Radiol 2000; 29(11):640–5.

39. Pierre-Jerome C, Moncayo V, Terk MR. MRI of the Achilles tendon: a comprehensive review of the anatomy, biomechanics, and imaging of overuse tendinopathies. Acta Radiol 2010;51(4):438–54.

40. Bottger BA, Schweitzer ME, El-Noueam KI, et al. MR imaging of the normal and abnormal retrocalcaneal bursae. AJR Am J Roentgenol 1998;170(5):1239–41.

41. Rosenberg ZS, Beltran J, Bencardino JT. From the RSNA Refresher Courses. Radiological Society of North America. MR imaging of the ankle and foot. Radiographics 2000;20 Spec No:S153–179.

42. Weinstable R, Stiskal M, Neuhold A, et al. Classifying calcaneal tendon injury according to MR findings. J Bone Joint Surg [Br] 1991;73:683–5.

43. Hartgerink P, Fessell DP, Jacobson JA, et al. Full- versus partial-thickness Achilles tendon tears: sonographic accuracy and characterization in 26 cases with surgical correlation. Radiology 2001;220(2):406–12.

44. Gärdin A, Bruno J, Movin T, et al. Magnetic resonance signal, rather than tendon volume, correlates to pain and functional impairment in chronic Achilles tendinopathy. Acta Radiol 2006;47(7):718–24.

45. Koulouris G, Connell D. Hamstring muscle complex: an imaging review. Radiographics 2005;25:571–86.

46. Agre JC. Hamstring injuries. Proposed aetiological factors, prevention, and treatment. Sports Med 1985;2(1):21–33.

47. Bencardino JT, Mellado JM. Hamstring injuries of the hip. Magn Reson Imaging Clin N Am 2005;13(4):677–90.

48. Takami H, Takahashi S, Ando M. Late sciatic nerve palsy following avulsion of the biceps femoris muscle from the ischial tuberosity. Arch Orthop Trauma Surg 2000; 120(5-6):352–4.

49. Beltran L, Ghazikhanian V, Padron M, et al. The proximal hamstring muscle-tendon-bone unit: a review of the normal anatomy, biomechanics, and pathophysiology. Eur J Radiol 2011. [Epub ahead of print].

50. De Smet A, Best T. MR Imaging of the distribution and location of acute hamstring injuries in athletes. AJR 2000;174:393–9.

51. Connell D, Schneider-Kolsky M, Hoving J. Longitudinal study comparing sonographic and MRI assessments of acute and healing hamstring injuries. AJR 2004;183:975–84.

52. Stevens M, El-Khoury G, Kathol M, et al. Imaging features of avulsion injuries. Radiographics 1999;19:655–72.

53. Koulouris G, Connell D. Evaluation of the hamstring muscle complex following acute injury. Skeletal Radiol 2003;32(10):582–9.

54. Palmer WE, Kuong SJ, Elmadbouh HM. MR imaging of myotendinous strain. AJR 1999;173(3):703–9.

55. Slavotinek J, Verrall G, Fon G. Hamstring injury in athletes: using MR imaging measurements to compare extent of muscle injury with amount of time lost from competition. AJR 2002;179:1621–28.

56. Stoller D. Magnetic resonance imaging in orthopaedics and sports medicine. Lippincott Williams and Wilkins; 2007.

57. Amendola A, Rorabeck Ch, Vellett D, et al. The use of magnetic resonance imaging in exertional compartment syndromes. Am J Sports Med 1990;18(1):29–34.

58. Gaeta M, Minutoli F, Mazziotti S, et al. Diagnostic imaging in athletes with chronic lower leg pain. AJR 2008;191(5):1412–9.

59. Verleisdonk EJ, van Gils A, van der Werken C. The diagnostic value of MRI scans for the diagnosis of chronic exertional compartment syndrome of the lower leg. Skeletal Radiol 2001;30(6): 321–5.

60. Eskelin MK, Lotjonen JM, Mantysaari MJ. Chronic exertional compartment syndrome: MR imaging at 0.1 T compared with tissue pressure measurement. Radiology 1998;206:333–7.

61. Van den Brand JG, Nelson T, Verleisdonk EJ, et al. The diagnostic value of intracompartmental pressure measurement, magnetic resonance imaging, and near infrared spectroscopy in chronic exertional compartment syndrome: a prospective study in 50 patients. Am J Sports Med 2005;33(5):699–704.

62. Lauder TD, Stuart MJ, Amrami KK, et al. Exertional compartment syndrome and the role of magnetic resonance imaging. Am J Phys Med Rehabil 2002; 81(4):315–9.

63. Andreisek G, White LM, Sussman MS, et al. T2* weighted and arterial spin labeling MRI of calf muscles in healthy volunteers and patients with chronic exertional compartment syndrome: preliminary experience. AJR 2009;193(4):W327–33.
64. Litwiller DV, Amrami KK, Dahm DL, et al. Chronic exertional compartment syndrome of the lower extremities: improved screening using a novel dual birdcage coil and in-scanner exercise protocol. Skeletal Radiol 2007;36(11):1067–75.
65. Moeyersoons JP, Martens M. Chronic exertional compartment syndrome: diagnosis and management. Acta Orthop Belg 2009;58(1):23–7.
66. Mellado JM, Perez del Palomar L. Muscle hernias of the lower leg: MRI findings. Skeletal Radiol 1999;28(8):465–9.
67. Yao L, Sinha U. Imaging the microcirculatory proton fraction of muscle with diffusion-weighted echo-planar imaging. Acad Radiol 2000;7(1):27–32.
68. Anil G, Kiang-Hiong T, Tse-Chiang H, et al. Dynamic computed tomography angiography: role in the evaluation of popliteal artery entrapment syndrome. Cardiovasc Intervent Radiol 2010;34(2):259–70.
69. Love JW, Whelan TJ. Popliteal artery entrapment syndrome. Am J Surg 1965;109: 620–4.
70. Rich NM, Collins GJ Jr, McDonald PT, et al. Popliteal vascular entrapment: its increasing interest. Arch Surg 1979;114:1377–84.
71. Macedo T, Johnson C, Hallet Jr J, et al. Popliteal artery entrapment syndrome: role of imaging in the diagnosis. Am J Radiol 2003;181:1259–65.
72. Kukreja K, Scagnelli T, Narayanan G, et al. Role of angiography in popliteal artery entrapment syndrome. Diagn Interv Radiol 2009;15:57–60.
73. Wright L, Matchett W, Cruz C, et al. Popliteal artery disease: diagnosis and treatment. Radiographics 2004;24:467–79.
74. Elias D, White L, Rubenstein J, et al. Clinical evaluation and MR imaging features of popliteal artery entrapment and cystic adventitial disease. Am J Radiol 2003;180: 627–32.

The Female Athlete Triad

Jay F. Deimel, MD[a], Bradley J. Dunlap, MD[b,c],*

KEYWORDS

- Sports • Athlete • Triad • Female • Osteopenia

The Triad Consensus Conference in 1992, conducted by the American College of Sports Medicine (ACSM) task force, originally defined the "female athlete triad" as disordered eating, amenorrhea, and osteoporosis. Since that time, there have been many national and international task forces and health initiatives active in this field as the number of women athletes has continued to grow. Further investigation has lead to the current definition of the "female athlete triad": low energy availability (with or without eating disorders), menstrual dysfunction, and altered bone mineral density (BMD).[1] This new position stand emphasizes efforts to research the underlying causes of this syndrome, as well as highlights the role of low energy availability as the key disorder among the triad.[2] It is important to note that a vast minority of athletes diagnosed with this syndrome actually manifests all three components to the same degree simultaneously.[3–5] Rather, the "triad" is best understood as a continuum ranging from health to disease of each disorder: energy availability, menstrual function, and bone density (**Fig. 1**). At any one time, affected athletes move between the points at varying rates according to their individual experience.[2] Because of the dire consequences associated with both the physical and mental health of the athlete affected by the triad, preventative measures are crucial to curbing the progression of this multifaceted syndrome.

PREVALENCE

In athletes, the prevalence of low energy availability, menstrual dysfunction, and altered BMD demonstrates marked variability.[6] In a study from 2006, Nichols and colleagues[4] examined the prevalence of the triad of disorders among 170 high school athletes from 8 different sports. Two athletes met the criteria for all 3 components and 10 females met the criteria for 2 components. Menstrual dysfunction, low BMD, and

The authors have nothing to disclose.

[a] Section of Orthopaedic Surgery and Rehabilitation Medicine, University of Chicago Medical Center, 5841 South Maryland Avenue, MC 3079, Chicago, IL 60637, USA

[b] Department of Orthopaedic Surgery, NorthShore University HealthSystem, 1000 Central Street, Suite 880, Evanston, IL 60201, USA

[c] Section of Orthopaedic Surgery and Rehabilitation Medicine, University of Chicago Pritzker School of Medicine, 924 East 57th Street, Suite 104, Chicago, IL 60637-5415, USA

* Corresponding author. Department of Orthopaedic Surgery, NorthShore University HealthSystem, 1000 Central Street, Suite 880, Evanston, IL 60201.

E-mail address: bdunlap@northshore.org

Clin Sports Med 31 (2012) 247–254

doi:10.1016/j.csm.2011.09.007

0278-5919/12/$ – see front matter © 2012 Elsevier Inc. All rights reserved.

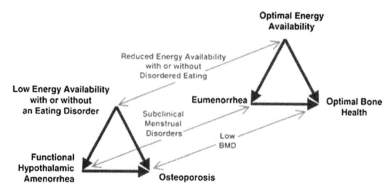

Fig. 1. The female athlete triad. (*From* Nattiv A, Loucks AB, Manore MM, et al. American College of Sports Medicine position stand. The female athlete triad. Med Sci Sports Exerc 2007;39(10):1868; with permission.)

disordered eating accounted for 23.5%, 21.8%, and 18.2%, respectively. Specifically, prevalence estimates of disordered eating among high school and collegiate athletes ranges from 15% to 62%[7,8] compared to 13% to 20% in the general adolescent female population. Additionally, research regarding the prevalence of menstrual dysfunction among athletes remains ambiguous, with estimates ranging between 3.4% and 66%.[4]

Possible explanations of the wide variability of the prevalence of the above triad components include different assessment methodologies between studies and the failure to abide by strict definable study characteristics. The passage of Title IX by Congress has also played an indirect role in regard to the prevalence of female athletes diagnosed with the triad. With its implementation in 1972, Title IX sought to ensure an equal opportunity for women in high school and intercollegiate athletics.[1,9] Since the onset of the passage, high school female athletics has continued to grow by leaps and bounds, including an approximate 4-fold increase to over 3 million active participants today. In the face of this dynamic growth in conjunction with the stressed ideals of perfection, winning, and body image comes the realization that the risk of the female athlete developing this syndrome is likely to increase.

ETIOLOGY

It has been theorized that the root of this syndrome begins with low energy availability.[3] The female athlete, seeking an improved body image to enhance athletic prowess, begins to restrict caloric intake. This restrictive dieting behavior then progresses, eventually predisposing the athlete to menstrual irregularity and decreased BMD.[9] Often, energy availability fluctuates daily, with direct and/or indirect effects on menstrual function and BMD that are realized months to years later.[1]

RISK FACTORS

Athletes at greatest risk for developing the Female Athlete Triad are those who restrict caloric intake, exercise for extended periods, and have vegetarian diets.[10] Specifically, athletes who develop abnormal eating behaviors may be predisposed based upon various social and/or environmental factors including psychological issues, low self-esteem, abuse, genetics, and family dysfunction.[1,11] Injury and an earlier commitment to sport-specific training are additional risk factors for the development of low energy availability.[12] Specifically, risk factors associated with development of stress fractures within this population include low BMD, menstrual dysfunction, dietary insufficiency, and genetic inheritance, among others.[13]

ENERGY AVAILABILITY

Energy availability is accurately defined as the dietary energy within the body after exercise training is completed; or simply total dietary energy minus exhausted exercise energy. The 2007 ACSM position stand repeatedly emphasizes the notion of a spectrum of abnormal eating behaviors, ranging from the broad category of low energy availability to poor eating habits and eating disorders.[1] Although low energy availability is synonymous with disordered eating, it is possible to occur free of any abnormal eating behavior. An athlete may fail to keep up with her energy requirements secondary to a rigorous daily routine and/or poor nutritional habit.[14] When energy availability falls below a critical threshold, normal physiological mechanisms are disrupted: namely, cellular maintenance, growth, and reproduction.[1,11]

Athletes can alter energy availability by either increasing energy expenditure or decreasing energy intake. Ways in which energy intake is decreased involve purging, fasting, use of diet pills, laxatives, and diuretics.[2] Current research has shown the prevalence of disordered eating, include a varied subset of eating disorders, to span between 1% and 62% in female athletes.[4] Eating disorders are defined as a clinical mental disorder also associated with other psychiatric issues. Two of the most common types of eating disorders found within athletes are anorexia nervosa and bulimia nervosa. Anorexia is defined as a clinical eating disorder wherein a person engages in restrictive eating behavior as he or she views himself or herself as being overweight despite weighing more than 15% below ideal body weight for age and height. On the other hand, an individual diagnosed with bulimia repeats a cycle of overeating then purging while often maintaining a normal weight for body habitus.[1]

Research suggests that there is ideally no single cause regarding the development of eating disorders among athletes. Instead, its presence is most likely multi-factorial, with various environmental, physiological, and cultural components. The ideal that the intense pressure associated with various athletic activities may incite the development of an eating disorder in athletes who are psychologically vulnerable is a continued topic of conversation.[14]

MENSTRUAL DYSFUNCTION

Topics present within this category of the Female Athlete Triad include anovulation, primary amenorrhea, secondary amenorrhea, oligomenorrhea, and luteal suppression. Before addressing these topics, it is important to define "normal." Eumenorrhea refers to menstrual cycles occurring at intervals near the mean interval for adult women (typically 28 ± 7 days). Within the general premenopausal adult female population, the incidence of menstrual dysfunction ranges fluctuates between 2% and 5%.[1] In comparison, approximately 6% to 79% of female athletes are said to experience menstrual dysfunction.[3]

Amenorrhea refers to the absence of menstrual cycles lasting longer than 3 months. Amenorrhea occurring after menarche is termed secondary amenorrhea, while a delay in the age of menarche is defined as primary amenorrhea.[6] Anovulation is defined as a menstrual cycle without ovulation. Oligomenorrhea denotes menstrual cycles longer than 35 days. The prevalence of oligomenorrhea in female athletes has been reported to be noticeably higher than in the general population, encompassing roughly 21% to 40% in sport-specific domains.[14]

As often the initiating factor of the triad, low energy availability induces a hypometabolic state. Strenuous training alone has not been shown to alter menstrual cycles; it is necessary for dietary restriction to occur.[15] In a study by Loucks and Thuma,[16] it was decided that the energy threshold at which menstrual dysfunction is likely to occur is approximately 30 kcal/kg lean body mass per day. This "energy deficit" theory describes the induction of menstrual irregularities secondary to an imbalance in the body's natural neuroendocrine function, specifically the impact on the hypothalamic-pituitary-adrenal axis. Disruption of the body's normal homeostatic mechanisms leads to the development of significant health consequences, including infertility, decreased immune function, and decreased BMD.

BONE MINERAL DENSITY

The last component of the triad is also best described as a spectrum encompassing optimum bone health, low bone density, and osteoporosis. Currently, bone strength is measured with dual-energy x-ray absorptiometry (DEXA), which specifically looks at one bone strength component—BMD. Other components play important roles when defining bone strength, specifically bone quality and bone mineral content. The dynamic process of bone turnover produced by osteoclasts (bone remodeling) and osteoblasts (bone formation) contributes to one's overall bone quality.[14] In the clinical setting at present, DEXA testing functions as the most accepted quantitative value in determining a patient's BMD and associated clinical implications. There has been increased emphasis over the past 10 years on the utilization of Z-scores (age- and gender-matched controls) instead of T-scores (30-year-old adult controls).[14] Traditionally, T-scores have been used to diagnose osteoporosis and to predict postmenopausal fracture risk. When discussing bone health in premenopausal women and teens, the International Society for Clinical Densitometry (ISCD) has moved away from the use of T-scores as an assessment of BMD. T-scores better serve to highlight the disparity in BMD between postmenopausal females and 30-year-old female control subjects. Considering the BMD of teens and young children, there would theoretically be an increase in diagnosis of osteopenia within this population if T-scores were used as peak bone density may have not yet been achieved. In regard to the triad, the ISCD has now championed the use of the Z-score, in which teens and young adults are compared to sex- and age-matched controls.[14] The ACSM defines osteopenia, or low BMD, to include a history stress fractures, hypoestrogenism, dietary imbalance along with a Z-score between −1.0 and −2.0.[1] Osteoporosis (Z-score ≤−2.0) is defined by the ACSM as a skeletal disorder with low bone strength predisposing one to an increased risk for fracture. Recently, the ISCD has altered this ACSM terminology by recommending Z-scores below −2.0 in premenopausal women be termed "low bone density below the expected range for age" and "low bone density for chronological age" in affected children.[1]

A female athlete's BMD is best described as a single snapshot of her cumulative bone health at any point in time based on many interrelated variables, namely energy availability, menstrual function, and genetic influence.[1] It is important for an athlete's BMD to be charted over time, so that she is informed of her trend and can attempt to make necessary changes as deviations arise. Since the majority of peak bone mass is accrued in childhood and adolescence, it is vital that at-risk athletes be identified in an attempt to prevent chronic poor bone health.[2] In fact, it is possible for premenopausal women who become amenorrheic, oligomenorrheic, or postmenopausal to lose approximately 2% of their BMD per year.

Average Total Bone Mineral Density By Sport

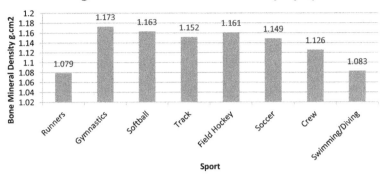

Fig. 2. Average bone mineral density among collegiate female athletes by sport. (*Data from* Mudd LM, Fornetti W, Pivarnik JM. Bone mineral density in collegiate female athletes: comparisons among sports. J Athl Train 2007;42:403–8.)

The prevalence of low bone density in athletes also is highly variable due to variations in definable parameters and the cost associated with diagnostic modalities. The presence of osteopenia in female athletes ranges from 22% to 50%.[17] However, female athletes in weight-bearing sports such as basketball and volleyball have a nearly 15% higher BMD than nonathletes. A recent study looking at average BMD in collegiate athletes across a number of sports found that runners had the lowest BMD of all sports investigated (**Fig. 2**).[18] The protective effect of weight bearing can be eliminated in athletes affected by other components of the triad. The development of stress fractures in athletes diagnosed with low BMD and menstrual dysfunction may approach a rate of 17%.[19] Cobb and colleagues analyzed the interaction of disordered eating, menstrual irregularity, and BMD among 91 competitive long-distance runners (ages 18 to 25) and discovered 6% of the amenorrheic group had spine BMD values termed "osteoporotic" with another 48% classified as "osteopenic."[17]

The etiology of this third triad component can be attributed in large part to the female's hypoestrogenic state. Within this framework, the female athlete demonstrates accelerated bone resorption due to the lack of the suppressive effect of estrogen on osteoclast activity. It is believed that other factors including low energy availability also play a significant role in the development of low BMD in female athletes.[14]

EVALUATION

Appropriate screening in at-risk athletes should take place during preparticipation exams or during annual health check-ups. Any long distance runner with recurrent leg pain, or under high suspicion for a stress fracture, should also undergo similar evaluation. The physician should have a firm understanding of all components of the triad, their unique interrelationships, and the entire spectrum from health to illness each component embodies.[1] It is both prudent and recommended to test an athlete for all triad components if she presents with a diagnosis of one.

Trainers, coaches, and parents are often the first to witness an athlete's abnormal psychological and behavioral characteristics. Examples include increased anxiety, unnecessary dieting, being "too critical," compulsiveness regarding exercise, social withdrawal, binge eating, substance abuse, and increased agitation. Therefore, a high index of suspicion must exist on the physician's part when dealing with athletes presenting with altered eating habits/behaviors or multiple physical complaints.[2] Even in the absence of a clinical diagnosis of anorexia or bulimia, the concern regarding abnormal types of eating behaviors remains heightened as this scenario can lead to low energy availability.

Pertinent components of the medical history include energy intake, dietary practices, weight fluctuations, and eating habits. The physician should also elicit a complete menstrual history including onset of menarche and current menstrual status. Sport-specific inquiries should include the number of training hours per day, number of sports played, and prior history of stress fracture/injury. An athlete with a history of disordered eating should be referred to a mental health practitioner for further workup.

Each visit should include a set of vitals (height, weight, blood pressure) along with BMI calculation and current menstrual status.[1] Physical exam findings that may be apparent in a patient effected by this triad include parotid gland enlargement, lanugo hair, acrocyanosis of the hands/feet, and bradycardia. Sexual maturity should be documented with Tanner staging. Pelvic examination may reveal vaginal atrophy if hypoestrogenism is present.[20]

A standard battery of laboratory tests should be obtained if clinical suspicion of one component of the triad is present. Specifically, a complete blood count with differential, complete metabolic panel, erythrocyte sedimentation rate, thyroid function tests, and urinalysis should be a part of the standard assessment.[14] Other more advanced tests include urine electrolytes (which may be low from recurrent vomiting), salivary amylase (which may be increased from vomiting), stool guaic (in cases of laxative abuse), and an electrocardiogram (assess for arrhythmias and prolonged QT interval). Evaluation for amenorrhea should consist of the following: pregnancy test, levels of follicle-stimulating hormone (FSH) and luteinizing hormone (LH), prolactin measurement, and a thyroid stimulating hormone test to assess for thyroid disease.[1] Evaluation by a reproductive specialist should be performed if an athlete's menses has not been restored within 3 to 6 months after initiation of treatment.

The ACSM recommends a baseline DEXA test should occur in an athlete with evidence of greater than 6 months of amenorrhea, oligomenorrhea, and/or disordered eating. A history of stress fractures should also prompt the physician to order a DEXA test. A diagnosis of low BMD or osteoporosis is formulated from the lowest Z-score from the spine or hip.

PREVENTION AND TREATMENT

Optimum treatment for those athletes diagnosed with the Female Athlete Triad must include a multidisciplinary team approach to maximize therapeutic effectiveness. This specialist-oriented team should consist of the following individuals: health care providers, mental-health practitioners, dieticians, coaches, parents, athletic trainers, exercise physiologist, etc. Although the primary emphasis is on prevention, each of the above individuals has the ability to impact the treatment plan of an affected athlete. Education originating within the school system on triad-specific components is critical to establishing a healthy awareness of the Female Athlete Triad. Young athletes should be alerted to the significant health risks of low BMD, menstrual dysfunction, and poor overall energy availability. Within the competitive arena, coaches should emphasize the benefits of proper nutrition in relation to the attainment of athletic achievements.

After a comprehensive treatment plan has been formulated, it is necessary for the treating physician along with the multidisciplinary team to determine whether an athlete may continue to train and participate in sport competitively. The athlete must comply with all treatment strategies, be closely monitored by a physician, place importance on treatment over training, and take steps to modify training (intensity, duration, type). If the athlete chooses to not accept treatment, breaks the contract, or does not show steady progression in weight gain, then the athlete must be removed from competition.[1]

The first aim of therapy focuses on energy availability. Specifically, it is essential to create an "energy positive" dietary environment by increasing intake, reducing energy expenditure, or a combination of the 2.[1] This increase in energy availability then translates into increased BMD and restoration of menstrual function.[20] For example, increases in BMD of nearly 5% per year have correlated with increases in body weight in amenorrheic athletes.[17] Any athlete presenting with signs and symptoms of disordered eating should be referred to nutritional counseling. The dietitian should estimate an athlete's daily energy availability through the use of a food diary. Bone-building supplements (vitamin D, calcium) should be administered.

The overall treatment goals for athletes presenting with disordered eating remain the following: improve nutritional status, modify unhealthy thoughts, and normalize eating behavior. Treatment success is intimately linked with the development of trustworthy relationships between athlete and care provider. Other forms of nonpharmacological therapy include individual psychotherapy, cognitive-behavioral therapy, and group therapy.[1]

Pharmacological therapy may help to serve as a useful adjunct in affected patients. Antidepressants are often prescribed by mental-health practitioners in patients exhibiting certain mental disorders and/or abnormal eating behaviors (ie, bulimia, anorexia). However, health practitioners must realize that hormone replacement therapy (HRT) and/or oral contraceptives (OCP) do not address the underlying pathological mechanisms of bone formation and health. Therefore, pharmacological treatment alone will not serve to restore age-appropriate BMD.[17] OCP agents are recommended in athletes older than 16 years with continued BMD decline in an effort to minimize further bone loss. Bisphosphonates, while approved for treatment of postmenopausal osteoporosis, are not recommended in the young athlete due to an overall lack of proven efficacy in this population, as well as concerns for potential harmful fetal effects.

SUMMARY

The Female Athlete Triad poses serious health risks, both short and long term, to the overall well-being of affected individuals. Sustained low energy availability can impair health, causing many medical complications within the skeletal, endocrine, cardiovascular, reproductive, and central nervous systems.[1] With the surge of females participating in athletics within the past 10 to 15 years, it is both conceivable and likely that the prevalence of this syndrome will continue to grow. Therefore, it is imperative that appropriate screening and diagnostic measures are enacted by a multidisciplinary team of health care providers, counselors, teachers, and dieticians in order to provide the proper care to affected athletes. Initial awareness should take place within the educational confines of elementary and high schools. Screening for female athletes exhibiting risk factors for the triad should also take place at the time of sports physicals. If one component of the triad is identified, the clinician should take the time to effectively workup the other 2. Treatment for each component of the triad includes both pharmacological and nonpharmacological measures, with emphasis placed upon increased energy availability and overall improved nutritional health. Using this all-encompassing type of approach, sports medicine practitioners should feel empowered to continue to promote the lifelong well-being of female athletes in the years to come.

REFERENCES

1. Nattiv A, Loucks AB, Manore MM, et al. American College of Sports Medicine. Position Stand: the female athlete triad. Med Sci Sports Exerc 2007;39:1867–82.
2. Lebrun CM. The Female Athlete Triad: what's a doctor to do? Curr Sports Med Rep 2007;6:397–404.
3. Beals KA, Hill AK. The prevalence of disordered eating, menstrual dysfunction, and low bone mineral density among US collegiate athletes. Int J Sports Nutr Exerc Metab 2006;16:1–23.
4. Nichols JF, Rauh MJ, Lawson MJ, et al. Prevalence of the female athlete triad syndrome among high school athletes. Arch Pediatr Adolesc Med 2006;160: 137–42.
5. Torstveit MK, Sundgot-Borgen J. The female athlete triad exists in both elite athletes and controls. Med Sci Sports Exerc 2005;37:1449–59.
6. Nichols DL, Sanborn CF. Female athlete and bone. In: Nutrition for Sport and Exercise. Gaithersburg (MD): Aspen Publishing; 1998. p. 205–15.
7. Johnson C, Powers PS, Dick R. Athletes and eating disorders: the National Collegiate Athletic Association study. Int J Eating Disord 1999;26:179–88.
8. Beals KA, Manore MM. Disorders of the female athlete triad among collegiate athletes. Int J Sports Nutr Exerc Metab 2002;12:281–93.
9. Hoch AZ, Pajewski NM, Moraski LA, et al. Prevalence of the Female Athlete Triad in high school athletes and sedentary students. Clin J Sports Med 2009;19: 421–8.
10. Manore MM. Nutritional needs of the female athlete. Clin J Sports Med 1999;18: 549–63.
11. Witkop CT, Warren MP. Understanding the spectrum of the Female Athlete Triad. Am Coll Obstet Gynecol 2010;116:1444–8.
12. Sundgot-Borgen J. Risk and trigger factors for the development of eating disorders in female elite athletes. Med Sci Sports Exerc 1994;26:414–9.
13. Boden BP, Osbahr DC. High-risk stress fractures: evaluation and treatment. J Am Acad Orthop Surg 2000;8:344–53.
14. Beals KA, Meyer NL. Female Athlete Triad update. Clin Sports Med 2007;26:69–89.
15. Williams NI, Helmreich DL, Parfitt DB, et al. Evidence for a causal role of low energy availability in the induction of menstrual cycle disturbances during strenuous exercise training. J Clin Endocrinol Metab 2001;86:5184–93.
16. Loucks AB, Thuma JR. Luteinizing hormone pulsatility is disrupted at a threshold of energy availability in regularly menstruating women. J Clin Endocrinol Metab 2003; 88:297–311.
17. Cobb KL, Bachrach LK, Greendale G, et al. Disordered eating, menstrual irregularity, and bone mineral density in female runners. Med Sci Sports Exerc 2002;711–9.
18. Mudd LM, Fornetti W, Pivarnik JM. Bone mineral density in collegiate female athletes: comparisons among sports. J Athletic Train 2007;42:403–8.
19. Torstveit MK, Sundgot-Borgen J. The female athlete triad: are elite athletes at increased risk? Med Sci Sports Exerc 2005;37:184–93.
20. Mendelsohn FA, Warren MP. Anorexia, bulimia, and the female athlete triad: evaluation and management. J Clin Endocrinol Metab 2010;39:155–67.

Muscle Soreness and Delayed-Onset Muscle Soreness

Paul B. Lewis, MD, MS[a],*, Deana Ruby, APN, ACNP-BC[b],
Charles A. Bush-Joseph, MD[b]

KEYWORDS
- Muscle soreness • DOMS • Delayed-onset • Muscle ache
- Stiffness

The novice and elite athlete is familiar with the postexercise muscle discomfort known as delayed-onset muscle soreness (DOMS) after unfamiliar exercises. While common in occurrence, most patients will self-treat the condition unless symptoms are progressive in nature. The sports medicine clinician needs to maintain this diagnosis among their active differential diagnoses. Associated symptomology of muscle soreness can be quite debilitating and the presentation of this phenomenon is as diverse as the population that experiences it.

Immediate or delayed-onset muscle soreness with a nonuniform intramuscular distribution may portray itself as a nonmuscular injury with an unrecalled or vague traumatic event. The prudent clinician is to base their advisory guidance, medical management and/or surgical treatments on sound medical and/or surgical principles. The purpose of this communication is to describe the clinical presentation, cellular mechanisms, preventative measures, and management options related to muscle soreness and DOMS for the sports medicine clinician.

CLINICAL PRESENTATION

Muscle soreness is classified as a type I muscle strain[1] and refers to the immediate soreness perceived by the athlete while or immediately after participating in exercises. Muscle soreness presents with muscle stiffness, aching pain, and/or muscular tenderness. These symptoms are experienced for only hours and are relatively transient compared to those of DOMS. The symptomatology of DOMS shares similar

The authors have nothing to disclose.
a Department of Diagnostic Radiology & Nuclear Medicine, Rush University Medical Center, 1653 West Congress Parkway, Chicago, IL 60612, USA
b Department of Orthopedic Surgery, Rush University Medical Center, Third Floor, 1611 West Harrison Street, Chicago, IL 60612, USA
* Corresponding author.
E-mail address: paul_lewis@rsh.net

Clin Sports Med 31 (2012) 255–262
doi:10.1016/j.csm.2011.09.009
0278-5919/12/$ – see front matter © 2012 Elsevier Inc. All rights reserved.

quality and intensity to that of immediate exercise-induced muscle soreness but symptom onset is at about 24 hours after the athlete has completed their exercise.[2,3] In the ensuing days, the related symptoms peak within 72 hours and slowly resolve in 5 to 7 days.[2,3] While the presentation of these conditions differs temporally, there is a shared subtly that may lead one to the clinical question of more concerning pain generators (eg, stress fracture, ligamentous sprain, or tendon tear).

Muscle soreness may begin as a concerted area sensitive to passive manipulation and active movement.[4,5] This early perception may later be perceived as broad muscle soreness with focal points of tenderness referred from the active process within the musculotendinous junction.[6] This latter presentation is more ambiguous, and accordingly more concerning. The clinical responsibility is to discern DOMS from a non-muscular injury with an unrecalled or vague traumatic event (eg, ligamentous rupture, chondral defect, stress fracture). To do so, it requires an understanding of the characteristics of DOMS and competing diagnoses.

Clinically, focal exercise-induced soreness can be separated from a nonmuscular etiology with reproducible active and passive, weight-bearing and non–weight-bearing range of motion. Moreover, the clinician can use specific tests to the possible surrounding nonmuscular etiologies. Expanding the diagnostic thought process to include recent changes in workout intensity, exercise duration, and the individual's baseline exercise tolerance will further direct one toward or away from an etiology. Finally, consideration of new activities the patient may have performed is warranted, particularly in patients who were already well conditioned.

Independent of the patient's previous condition, there is an associated muscle weakness after an episode of acute or delayed muscular soreness.[5,7–11] This decline in muscular performance is intuitively related to the associated cell damage and subsequent inflammatory response.[12–14] The identified cellular damage related to unaccustomed exercise is loss of membrane integrity[15,16] and excitation-contraction coupling.[12,14] Restoration of muscle strength from the causative exercise may take up to 2 weeks to occur.[4] The delay in recovery has been attributed to the inflammatory cell infiltration and accumulation.[61,63] Clinically, the strength deficit and its duration deserve to be included when advising patients whom are considering beginning or increasing their exercise program.

Concurrently, as focus turns to "return to play" during or after the resolution of muscle soreness, the clinician is to remain grounded with injury risk factors that include but are not limited to subtle deficiencies in joint stabilization and cushioning,[17] gross coordination,[17,18] and, as above, strength.[12–14]

CELLULAR MECHANISMS

Paralleling the diverse population and clinical presentation of muscle soreness, there are 6 competing theories for the mechanism of DOMS: lactic acid accumulation,[19,20] muscle spasm,[21,22] microtrauma,[23–25] connective tissue damage,[25] inflammation,[5,9,26] and electrolytes and enzyme efflux.[19,27,28] While these 6 theories were presented independently from one another, the current consensus is that a single theory alone is insufficient to explain the process; instead, they work in concert.[19,20,29–31]

The mechanism of muscle soreness, immediate and delayed onset, begins at the time of exercise with strain on the muscle's functional unit—the sarcomere. Subsequent to breakdown of the functional unit, there is an intracellular accumulation of calcium, causing further degradation of the sarcomere. This intracellular damage increases the demands on surrounding connective tissue. Following this is an inflammatory response with recruitment of inflammatory cells and cytokines that potentiate the nerve endings and perception of pain. Passive manipulation and active movement alter intramuscular pressures and stimulate mechanoreceptor nerve endings, contributing to the perception of soreness.[19,20,29–31]

Explanation of disproportionate (nonuniform) exercise-induced soreness begins with the intramuscular architecture.[32–34] Each imposed stress on muscles (eg, concentric versus eccentric actions) recruits different branches of a structural, intramuscular organization. Demands on selected parts within muscle develop selective pathways for electrical activity, hypertrophy, and generation of forces.[35–41] The gross manifestation of this intramuscular architecture is the orientation and shape of muscle. Had such intramuscular architecture not existed, the gastrocnemius would be a homogeneous, uniform cylinder of muscle tissue between the tendons. The demanded contractions during unaccustomed exercises may overload underdeveloped muscle fibers and lead to cellular damage.[42–44] Subsequent inflammation remains specific to those posits of underdeveloped myocytes within that architecture.[5,9,26] Ultimately, this translates into focal points of tenderness overlying typical locations of long bone stress fractures or superficial to a ligament's site of insertion.

PREVENTIVE MEASURES

Effective prevention of muscle soreness is difficult; it is a physiologic response to activity. The most effective prophylaxis of muscle soreness would be abstaining from prolonged, intense unfamiliar physical exercises. Identifying such activities before participating often carries a commensurate degree of difficulty. When such tasks are identified or anticipated however, there are inherent modalities—physical preparation, demand reduction and nutritional resources—can minimize anticipated muscle soreness.

Prevention of muscle soreness through stretching is supported by the rationale of viscoelastic and stress-relaxation behaviors of muscle.[20] The benefit of stretching, however, is marginal.[45,46] The 2011 Cochrane Database review by Herbert and colleagues[46] found the reduction of DOMS is maximized with stretching before and after activity.

Use of assistive devices may alleviate the demand on muscle fibers and decrease subsequent soreness.[47] When desired to maintain muscle demand and recruitment, the athlete is to be advised regarding nutritional supplements.

Carbohydrate and protein supplement drinks are seen to be most beneficial when consumed after, not prior to, muscle-damaging exercise activity.[48,49] In a sophisticated, double-blind study by Matsumoto and colleagues,[50] protein supplement surpassed the placebo drink in reducing muscle soreness and fatigue after prolonged physical exercise.

The use of supplements, assistive devices, and stretching is to be done cautiously and with a confirmation of understanding from the athlete on instructions. Additional preventative measures are also included next because of the crossover between prevention and symptom management.

SYMPTOM MANAGEMENT

Completing the physiological mechanism of muscle soreness is the only effective treatment. Each clinician is to approach the most compatible options for the athlete with a sound understanding of existing basic science that supports or refutes the selected modalities. The primary responsibility of the clinician is to prevent the athlete from injuring himself or herself with the chosen management(s).

The outcomes from clinical research on massage are too variable[28,51–55] to confidently support its gainful benefit; its use should be directed empirically by athlete perception. As suggested by Cheung and colleagues,[20] the variability of outcomes from massage are likely related to the variations in timing and methods of the studied tissue massage. Additionally, it is unclear if massage increases local blood flow to affected muscle.[56–58]

Recommendations of cryotherapy, vibration treatment, and nutriceutics (eg, pomegranate juice) carry the same degree of neutrality. Sample sizes, scheduling, and treatment administration have limited the value of studies of such methods.[59–70]

The rationale and outcomes of pharmaceutical intervention with nonsteroidal anti-inflammatory drugs (NSAIDs) are supported consistently and thus are recommended when provided with a reasonable guidance on the dangers[71] of their use. Clinically, NSAIDs decrease perceived muscle soreness associated with DOMS[72–77] but fail to impact the length or degree of muscle weakness.[72–77]

Further research is needed but supported in the use of mechanical lower extremity compression as it has been shown to reduce swelling and decrease perceived muscle soreness.[78] The same study by Kraemer and colleagues[78] showed continuous compression also allowed the maintenance of elbow range of motion and promotion of strength reconditioning.

The most effective, and highly recommended, modality to treat muscle soreness is continued exercise.[19,20,79] The basic principle supporting exercise is the increase in local blood flow and endorphin release it produces and its subsequent analgesic effects.[20,25,80] While effective, the athlete is more likely to cause muscular injury while exercising[81] and benefits diminish at the cessation of activity.

Surgical intervention[82] is not recommended as a prophylactic or treatment modality.

SUMMARY

Immediate and delayed-onset muscle soreness differ mainly in chronology of presentation. Both conditions share the same quality of pain, eliciting and relieving activities and a varying degree of functional deficits. There is no single mechanism for muscle soreness; instead, it is a culmination of 6 different mechanisms. The developing pathway of DOMS begins with microtrauma to muscles and then surrounding connective tissues. Microtrauma is then followed by an inflammatory process and subsequent shifts of fluid and electrolytes. Throughout the progression of these events, muscle spasms may be present, exacerbating the overall condition.

There are a multitude of modalities to manage the associated symptoms of immediate soreness and DOMS. Outcomes of each modality seem to be as diverse as the modalities themselves. The judicious use of NSAIDs and continued exercise are suggested to be the most reliable methods and recommended. This review article and each study cited, however, represent just one part of the clinician's decision-making process.[83] Careful affirmation of temporary deficits from muscle soreness is not to be taken lightly, nor is the advisement and medical management of muscle soreness prescribed by the clinician.

REFERENCES

1. Safran MR, Seaber AV, Garrett WE Jr. Warm-up and muscular injury prevention. An update. Sports Med 1989;8:239.
2. Byrnes WC, Clarkson PM. Delayed onset muscle soreness and training. Clin Sports Med 1986;5:605.
3. Ebbeling CB, Clarkson PM. Exercise-induced muscle damage and adaptation. Sports Med 1989;7:207.

4. Lieber RL, Friden J. Morphologic and mechanical basis of delayed-onset muscle soreness. J Am Acad Orthop Surg 2002;10:67.
5. MacIntyre DL, Reid WD, McKenzie DC. Delayed muscle soreness. The inflammatory response to muscle injury and its clinical implications. Sports Med 1995;20:24.
6. Gibson W, Arendt-Nielsen L, Graven-Nielsen T. Delayed onset muscle soreness at tendon-bone junction and muscle tissue is associated with facilitated referred pain. Exp Brain Res 2006;174:351.
7. Faulkner JA, Brooks SV, Opiteck JA. Injury to skeletal muscle fibers during contractions: conditions of occurrence and prevention. Phys Ther 1993;73:911.
8. MacIntyre DL, Reid WD, Lyster DM, et al. Presence of WBC, decreased strength, and delayed soreness in muscle after eccentric exercise. J Appl Physiol 1996;80:1006.
9. Paulsen G, Crameri R, Benestad HB, et al. Time course of leukocyte accumulation in human muscle after eccentric exercise. Med Sci Sports Exerc 2010;42:75.
10. Raastad T, Hallen J. Recovery of skeletal muscle contractility after high- and moderate-intensity strength exercise. Eur J Appl Physiol 2000;82:206.
11. Raastad T, Risoy BA, Benestad HB, et al. Temporal relation between leukocyte accumulation in muscles and halted recovery 10-20 h after strength exercise. J Appl Physiol 2003;95:2503.
12. Ingalls CP, Warren GL, Williams JH, et al. E-C coupling failure in mouse EDL muscle after in vivo eccentric contractions. J Appl Physiol 1998;85:58.
13. Louis E, Raue U, Yang Y, et al. Time course of proteolytic, cytokine, and myostatin gene expression after acute exercise in human skeletal muscle. J Appl Physiol 2007;103:1744.
14. Warren GL, Ingalls CP, Shah SJ, et al. Uncoupling of in vivo torque production from EMG in mouse muscles injured by eccentric contractions. J Physiol 1999; 515(Pt 2):609.
15. Brancaccio P, Maffulli N, Buonauro R, et al. Serum enzyme monitoring in sports medicine. Clin Sports Med 2008;27:1.
16. Byrnes WC, Clarkson PM, White JS, et al. Delayed onset muscle soreness following repeated bouts of downhill running. J Appl Physiol 1985;59:710.
17. Smith LL. Causes of delayed onset muscle soreness and the impact on athletic performance: a review. J Appl Sport Sci Res 1992;6:135.
18. Edgerton VR, Wolf SL, Levendowski DJ, et al. Theoretical basis for patterning EMG amplitudes to assess muscle dysfunction. Med Sci Sports Exerc 1996;28:744.
19. Armstrong RB. Mechanisms of exercise-induced delayed onset muscular soreness: a brief review. Med Sci Sports Exerc 1984;16:529.
20. Cheung K, Hume P, Maxwell L. Delayed onset muscle soreness: treatment strategies and performance factors. Sports Med 2003;33:145.
21. De Vries HA. Neuromuscular tension and its relief. J Assoc Phys Ment Rehabil 1962;16:86.
22. De Vries HA. Quantitative electromyographic investigation of the spasm theory of muscle pain. Am J Phys Med 1966;45:119.
23. Bobbert MF, Hollander AP, Huijing PA. Factors in delayed onset muscular soreness of man. Med Sci Sports Exerc 1986;18:75.
24. Friden J, Seger J, Ekblom B. Sublethal muscle fibre injuries after high-tension anaerobic exercise. Eur J Appl Physiol Occup Physiol 1988;57:360.
25. Hough T. Ergographic studies in muscular fatigue and soreness. J Boston Soc Med Sci 1900;5(3):81–92.
26. MacIntyre DL, Reid WD, Lyster DM, et al. Different effects of strenuous eccentric exercise on the accumulation of neutrophils in muscle in women and men. Eur J Appl Physiol 2000;81:47.

27. Gulick DT, Kimura IF. Delayed onset muscle soreness: what is it and how do we treat it? J Sport Rehab 1996;5:234.

28. Gulick DT, Kimura IF, Sitler M, et al. Various treatment techniques on signs and symptoms of delayed onset muscle soreness. J Athl Train 1996;31:145.

29. Armstrong RB. Initial events in exercise-induced muscular injury. Med Sci Sports Exerc 1990;22:429.

30. Smith LL. Acute inflammation: the underlying mechanism in delayed onset muscle soreness? Med Sci Sports Exerc 1991;23:542.

31. Weerakkody NS, Whitehead NP, Canny BJ, et al. Large-fiber mechanoreceptors contribute to muscle soreness after eccentric exercise. J Pain 2001;2:209.

32. Lieber RL, Friden J. Clinical significance of skeletal muscle architecture. Clin Orthop Relat Res 2001;(383):140–51.

33. Lieber RL, Friden J. Functional and clinical significance of skeletal muscle architecture. Muscle Nerve 2000;23:1647.

34. Noonan TJ, Garrett WE Jr. Injuries at the myotendinous junction. Clin Sports Med 1992;11:783.

35. Brown JM, Solomon C, Paton M. Further evidence of functional differentiation within biceps brachii. Electromyogr Clin Neurophysiol 1993;33:301.

36. Foley JM, Jayaraman RC, Prior BM, et al. MR measurements of muscle damage and adaptation after eccentric exercise. J Appl Physiol 1999;87:2311.

37. Levy AS, Kelly BT, Lintner SA, et al. Function of the long head of the biceps at the shoulder: electromyographic analysis. J Shoulder Elbow Surg 2001;10:250.

38. Meyer RA, Prior BM. Functional magnetic resonance imaging of muscle. Exerc Sport Sci Rev 2000;28:89.

39. Sakurai G, Ozaki J, Tomita Y, et al. Electromyographic analysis of shoulder joint function of the biceps brachii muscle during isometric contraction. Clin Orthop Relat Res 1998;(354):123–31.

40. Sarti MA, Monfort M, Fuster MA, et al. Muscle activity in upper and lower rectus abdominus during abdominal exercises. Arch Phys Med Rehabil 1996;77:1293.

41. Ward SR, Hentzen ER, Smallwood LH, et al. Rotator cuff muscle architecture: implications for glenohumeral stability. Clin Orthop Relat Res 2006;448:157.

42. Friden J, Lieber RL. Eccentric exercise-induced injuries to contractile and cytoskeletal muscle fibre components. Acta Physiol Scand 2001;171:321.

43. Lieber RL, Shah S, Friden J. Cytoskeletal disruption after eccentric contraction-induced muscle injury [review]. Clin Orthop Relat Res 2002;(403 Suppl):S90–9.

44. Patel TJ, Das R, Friden J, et al. Sarcomere strain and heterogeneity correlate with injury to frog skeletal muscle fiber bundles. J Appl Physiol 2004;97:1803.

45. Herbert RD, de Noronha M. Stretching to prevent or reduce muscle soreness after exercise. Cochrane Database Syst Rev 2007;7:CD004577.

46. Herbert RD, de Noronha M, Kamper SJ. Stretching to prevent or reduce muscle soreness after exercise. Cochrane Database Syst Rev 2011;7:CD004577.

47. Howatson G, Hough P, Pattison J, et al. Trekking poles reduce exercise-induced muscle injury during mountain walking. Med Sci Sports Exerc 2011;43(1):140–5.

48. Cockburn E, Stevenson E, Hayes PR, et al. Effect of milk-based carbohydrate-protein supplement timing on the attenuation of exercise-induced muscle damage. Appl Physiol Nutr Metab 2010;35(3):270–7.

49. McBrier NM, Vairo GL, Bagshaw D, et al. Cocoa-based protein and carbohydrate drink decreases perceived soreness after exhaustive aerobic exercise: a pragmatic preliminary analysis. J Strength Cond Res 2010;24(8):2203–10.

50. Matsumoto K, Koba T, Hamada K, et al. Branched-chain amino acid supplementation attenuates muscle soreness, muscle damage and inflammation during an intensive training program. J Sports Med Phys Fitness 2009;49:424.
51. Frey Law LA, Evans S, Knudtson J, et al. Massage reduces pain perception and hyperalgesia in experimental muscle pain: a randomized, controlled trial. J Pain 2008;9:714.
52. Hart JM, Swanik CB, Tierney RT. Effects of sport massage on limb girth and discomfort associated with eccentric exercise. J Athl Train 2005;40:181.
53. Isabell WK, Durrant E, Myrer W, et al. The effects of ice massage, ice massage with exercise, and exercise on the prevention and treatment of delayed onset muscle soreness. J Athl Train 1992;27:208.
54. Weber MD, Servedio FJ, Woodall WR. The effects of three modalities on delayed onset muscle soreness. J Orthop Sports Phys Ther 1994;20:236.
55. Zainuddin Z, Newton M, Sacco P, et al. Effects of massage on delayed-onset muscle soreness, swelling, and recovery of muscle function. J Athl Train 2005;40:174.
56. Cafarelli E, Flint F. The role of massage in preparation for and recovery from exercise. An overview. Sports Med 1992;14:1.
57. Hovind H, Nielsen SL. Effect of massage on blood flow in skeletal muscle. Scand J Rehabil Med 1974;6:74.
58. Tiidus PM. Manual massage and recovery of muscle function following exercise: a literature review. J Orthop Sports Phys Ther 1997;25:107.
59. Ayles S, Graven-Nielsen T, Gibson W. Vibration-induced afferent activity augments delayed onset muscle allodynia. J Pain 2011;12(8):884–91.
60. Bakhtiary AH, Safavi-Farokhi Z, Aminian-Far A. Influence of vibration on delayed onset of muscle soreness following eccentric exercise. Br J Sports Med 2007;41:145.
61. Connolly DA, McHugh MP, Padilla-Zakour OI, et al. Efficacy of a tart cherry juice blend in preventing the symptoms of muscle damage. Br J Sports Med 2006;40:679.
62. Denegar CR, Perrin DH. Effect of transcutaneous electrical nerve stimulation, cold, and a combination treatment on pain, decreased range of motion, and strength loss associated with delayed onset muscle soreness. J Athl Train 1992;27:200.
63. Lau WY, Nosaka K. Effect of vibration treatment on symptoms associated with eccentric exercise-induced muscle damage. Am J Phys Med Rehabil 2011;90(8): 648–57.
64. Raub W. From the National Institutes of Health. JAMA 1990;264:1086.
65. Rhea MR, Bunker D, Marin PJ, et al. Effect of iTonic whole-body vibration on delayed-onset muscle soreness among untrained individuals. J Strength Cond Res 2009;23:1677.
66. Rowsell GJ, Coutts AJ, Reaburn P, et al. Effect of post-match cold-water immersion on subsequent match running performance in junior soccer players during tournament play. J Sports Sci 2011;29(1):1–6.
67. Rowsell GJ, Coutts AJ, Reaburn P, et al. Effects of cold-water immersion on physical performance between successive matches in high-performance junior male soccer players. J Sports Sci 2009;27:565.
68. Trombold JR, Barnes JN, Critchley L, et al. Ellagitannin consumption improves strength recovery 2-3 d after eccentric exercise. Med Sci Sports Exerc 2010;42(3): 493–8.
69. Trombold JR, Reinfeld AS, Casler JR, et al. The effect of pomegranate juice supplementation on strength and soreness after eccentric exercise. J Strength Cond Res 2011;25(7):1782–8.
70. Weerakkody NS, Percival P, Hickey MW, et al. Effects of local pressure and vibration on muscle pain from eccentric exercise and hypertonic saline. Pain 2003;105:425.

71. Adams SS, Bough RG, Cliffe EE, et al. Some aspects of the pharmacology, metabolism, and toxicology of ibuprofen. I. Pharmacology and metabolism. Rheumatol Phys Med 1970;10:Suppl 10:9–26.
72. Cannavino CR, Abrams J, Palinkas LA, et al. Efficacy of transdermal ketoprofen for delayed onset muscle soreness. Clin J Sport Med 2003;13:200.
73. Donnelly AE, McCormick K, Maughan RJ, et al. Effects of a non-steroidal anti-inflammatory drug on delayed onset muscle soreness and indices of damage. Br J Sports Med 1988;22:35–8.
74. Dudley GA, Czerkawski J, Meinrod A, et al. Efficacy of naproxen sodium for exercise-induced dysfunction muscle injury and soreness. Clin J Sport Med 1997;7(1):3–10.
75. Francis KT, Hoobler T. Effects of aspirin on delayed muscle soreness. J Sports Med Phys Fitness 1987;27:333.
76. Hasson SM, Daniels JC, Divine JG, et al. Effect of ibuprofen use on muscle soreness, damage, and performance: a preliminary investigation. Med Sci Sports Exerc 1993;25:9.
77. Lecomte JM, Lacroix VJ, Montgomery DL. A randomized controlled trial of the effect of naproxen on delayed onset muscle soreness and muscle strength. Clin J Sport Med 1998;8:82.
78. Kraemer WJ, Bush JA, Wickham RB, et al. Influence of compression therapy on symptoms following soft tissue injury from maximal eccentric exercise. J Orthop Sports Phys Ther 2001;31:282.
79. Smith LL. Cause of delayed onset muscle soreness and the impact on athletic performance: a review. J Appl Sport Sci Res 1992;6:135.
80. Carlsson CA, Pellettieri L. A clinical view of pain physiology. Acta Chir Scand 1982;148:305.
81. Mair SD, Seaber AV, Glisson RR, et al. The role of fatigue in susceptibility to acute muscle strain injury. Am J Sports Med 1996;24:137.
82. Micklewright D. The effect of soft tissue release on delayed onset muscle soreness: a pilot study. Phys Ther Sport 2009;10:19.
83. Steves R. Appraising clinical studies: a commentary on the Zainuddin et al and Hart et al studies. J Athl Train 2005;40:186.

Hamstring Strains and Tears in the Athlete

Kashif Ali, MD, J. Martin Leland, MD*

KEYWORDS

- Hamstring • Strain • Tear • Rupture • Repair • Athlete
- Proximal hamstring rupture • Proximal hamstring repair

Acute and chronic hamstring injuries can be debilitating injuries in both professional athletes as well as those who participate in noncompetitive sports. In the elite athlete, hamstring injuries can cause prolonged absence from competition and are associated with a high recurrence rate.[1] As modern athletes push the limits of human endurance, as with ultramarathoners or collegiate athletes aspiring for the professional level, these types of injuries are bound to present themselves. Hamstring strains usually occur at the myotendinous junction (where force is concentrated) while an eccentric load is applied to the muscle.[2] This injury is common in sports that require sprinting, jumping, or quick acceleration or deceleration. The mainstay for treating low- to mid-grade strains has traditionally been conservative management, the goal of which is to restore the athlete back to his or her previous level of activity without predisposing them to future injury. This includes the RICE protocol (rest, ice, compression, elevation), activity modification, and gradual rehabilitation. Surgical management is rare and usually reserved for complete avulsion injuries either proximally off the ischial tuberosity or distally from the proximal fibula or tibia. Although studies on surgical management are few, the preliminary results show promising findings.[3–6]

ANATOMY

The hamstrings consist of 3 muscles: semimembranosus, semitendinosus, and biceps femoris (long and short heads). All 3 originate from a common point of origin on the ischial tuberosity. The anatomic origin of the semimembranosus tendon is the most lateral; the semitendinosus and long head of the biceps femoris form a conjoint tendon and originate medial to the origin of the semimembranosus.[1] The short head of the biceps originates along the lateral lip of the linea aspera and lateral intermuscular septum. The semitendinosus and semimembranosus both descend along the

Dr Leland is a consultant for Stryker.
Department of Orthopaedic Surgery, University of Chicago, 5841 South Maryland Avenue, MC 3079, Chicago, IL 60637, USA
* Corresponding author.
E-mail address: mleland@surgery.bsd.uchicago.edu

Clin Sports Med 31 (2012) 263–272
doi:10.1016/j.csm.2011.11.001
0278-5919/12/$ – see front matter © 2012 Elsevier Inc. All rights reserved.

medial portion of the thigh to insert on the pes anserinus and posteromedial portion of the tibia, respectively. The long and short heads of the biceps femoris attach to the fibular head as well as small contributions to the lateral collateral ligament and the lateral plateau of the tibia.[7] All of the hamstring muscles are innervated by the tibial portion of the sciatic nerve except for the short head of the biceps, which is innervated by the peroneal branch.

One factor that predisposes the hamstring muscles to injury is the fact that they cross both the hip and knee joints. This puts the muscle group at greater risk to be loaded eccentrically than muscles crossing only a single joint. Given this anatomic consideration, the hamstrings become extensors of the hip and flexors of the knee during the gait cycle.[7] According to anatomic studies, the musculotendinous junction extends over the entire length of the biceps femoris muscle making even midmuscle tears myotendinous injuries.[8]

DIAGNOSIS
History

Hamstring injuries usually are the result of sudden hip flexion with associated knee extension. These injuries are common in sprinters, football players, and water skiers. Patients report the acute onset of pain localized to the posterior thigh. In the acute setting, they are usually unable to continue participating in their chosen sport. In patients who have a complete rupture from the ischial tuberosity, pain can be localized to the proximal thigh with point tenderness at the ischial tubercle. However, proximal hamstring ruptures often are associated with distal semimembranosus strains, and these distal injuries may divert the attention away from the proximal rupture.

Patients with acute hamstring injuries usually will have pain with weight bearing and ambulate with a stiff-legged gait as a result of avoiding hip and knee flexion.[3] According to the literature, there is no agreed upon risk factors for the development of hamstring strains. However, most studies indicate that the previous hamstring injury increases the risk of reinjury.[9–12] This may be attributed to architectural changes at the cellular level after moderate to severe hamstring strains where scar tissue replaces normal muscle tissue.

Physical Examination

It is often difficult to determine the exact nature of the injury on examination given the deep location of the hamstring muscle group.[3] There usually is swelling localized to the posterior thigh with associated tenderness to palpation or induration along the hamstring muscle bellies. Often in more severe cases, an area of ecchymosis along the posterior thigh and knee can accompany these injuries (**Fig. 1**). Complete ruptures may present with a palpable defect within the muscle substance or proximally off the ischial tuberosity, which may or may not be felt on examination. In cases of severe injury, a wad of muscle may appear in the posterior thigh with muscle contraction.[2]

To fully examine the hamstrings, we prefer to examine patients in the prone position. Extending the knee may sometimes stimulate cramping and limit the examination.[2] Knee flexion strength is tested and compared with the contralateral side. In our experience, significant weakness of knee flexion strength in the prone position (30% strength or less in comparison with the uninjured limb) and significant posterior thigh/knee ecchymosis are usually indicative of an acute proximal hamstring rupture and warrants evaluation with more advanced imaging (magnetic resonance imaging [MRI]).

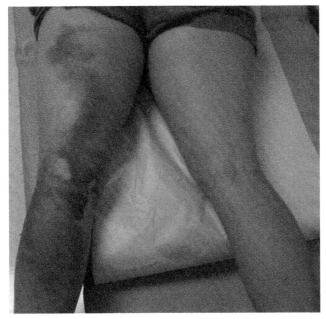

Fig. 1. Patient displaying extensive ecchymosis along the posterior thigh, knee, and calf after a complete proximal hamstring rupture.

Diagnostic Studies

As with any orthopaedic injury, plain films are the first diagnostic test when evaluating hamstring injuries. In most cases, radiographs will be negative for pathology. However, in the instance of severe injury or complete rupture, one may see a fleck of bone at the ischial tuberosity or an avulsion fracture.

Ultrasound scan can be used in the diagnosis of these injuries but does not give as much detail as more advanced imaging techniques. MRI has become crucial in determining the amount of soft tissue injury (**Fig. 2**). MRI is a useful tool for the orthopedist in determining complete versus partial rupture, number of tendons ruptures, and amount of retraction.[3] These variables may affect surgical decision making in certain patient populations. For most clinicians, the diagnosis of hamstring injury is made on history and physical examination. MRI serves as confirmation in most instances.

CLASSIFICATION

Muscle injuries can be classified as direct or indirect and are typically grouped into 3 categories according to severity.[13] Muscle strains are classified as indirect injuries that can be either incomplete or complete. Classically, strains are classified into 3 broad categories: grades I, II, and III. Grade I injuries occur with overstretching of the muscle with minimal loss of the structural integrity of the musculotendinous unit.[2] Grade II injuries are partial or incomplete tears. Grade III injuries, the most severe, constitute complete ruptures of the muscle either midsubstance or from the ischial tuberosity.

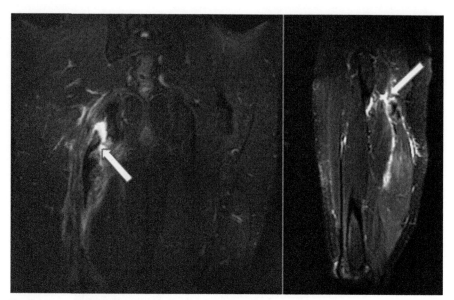

Fig. 2. Coronal (*left*) and saggital (*right*) MRI of acute proximal hamstring tendon rupture (*white arrows* depict tear).

TREATMENT
Nonoperative

The treatment of hamstring injuries remains a challenge for both athletes and clinicians, given their high incidence rate, slow healing, and persistent symptoms.[14] Although a few articles have been written regarding rehabilitation after hamstring strain, there has been no consensus on the best way to rehabilitate these injuries.[15–19]

In the acute setting, however, most agree that the standard treatment for hamstring strains has been initiating the RICE (rest, ice, compression, elevation) protocol. This limits the initial inflammatory response and helps control edema and hemorrhage. We recommend patients use ACE wrap as opposed to compression shorts so they can adjust the amount of compression according to their comfort level. Many advocate a gradual mobilization after the initial injury, which may allow for better regeneration, orientation, and alignment of the injured muscle fibers.[20,21] This gradual return to sport is usually made over a period of 4 to 6 weeks.[3] It is important to note that the nonoperative approach to treating hamstring injuries is individually tailored to the severity of injury. Those with extensive muscle and soft tissue damage may experience a prolonged recovery compared with those with a low-grade strain. Given this discrepancy, there is no set therapy algorithm for these injuries, rather a recovery program revolving around the patient's symptoms and pain level. In our experience, once patients are able to perform their daily activities as well as participate in their specific sport with little to no pain on a daily basis they are ready to return to competitive play. The postoperative protocol attached at the end of the article can be personalized and applied to the nonoperative treatment of hamstring strains as well.

The role of corticosteroids has also been studied in the treatment of hamstring injuries. Levine and Bergfeld [22] looked at 58 National Football League players with discrete hamstring strains with a palpable defect on examination. These players then received an intramuscular injection of corticosteroid and local anesthetic into the area of the defect. Although there were no controls for the study, they reported an average time to return to full practice was 7.6 days, and 49 players missed no game time. These results are promising; however, the potential side effect of injecting corticosteroids into injured muscles must be considered. The use of platelet-rich plasma is also becoming more popular among sports medicine physicians to treat a variety of injuries. Currently, no studies have looked at the direct effect of platelet-rich plasma on hamstring strains; however, a recent review of the literature by Taylor and colleagues[23] shows some promising results with other ligament and tendon injuries.

Returning to activity too soon may put patients at high risk for reinjury.[24] Given the high incidence of recurrence in hamstring injuries, some have tried to predict when elite athletes would be able to return to sport. One such study by Cohen and coworkers[25] looked at MRI correlation with return to play in professional football players. They determined those with isolated long head tears with less than 50% involvement had a rapid return to play, whereas those with multiple muscle injury and greater than 75% muscle involvement went on to have a more prolonged recovery and subsequently missed more games.

Operative

The surgical treatment of hamstring injuries is usually reserved for complete ruptures of the proximal hamstrings at their origin. According to Cohen and Bradley,[3] surgical management is recommended when 2 or 3 hamstrings are avulsed from the ischial tuberosity with greater than 2 cm of retraction. In 2002, Klingele and Sallay[4] reported the outcome of nonoperative treatment of 12 patients who had severe avulsion injuries to the proximal hamstring tendons. They concluded that there was persistent and significant functional impairment among patients with complete proximal rupture of the hamstring tendons, and this impairment was most profound during vigorous activities. In addition, a review of the literature by Harris and Griesser[6]

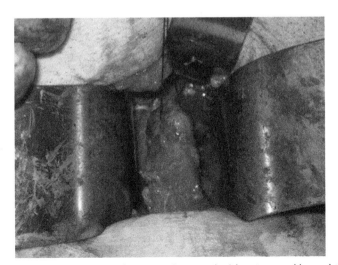

Fig. 3. The proximal hamstring tendon stump is tagged with suture and brought out of the wound.

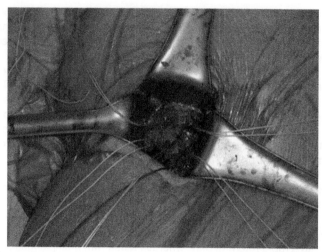

Fig. 4. Bioabsorbable suture anchors placed into the ischial tuberosity in an "X" configuration.

found that acute surgical repair had significantly better patient satisfaction, subjective outcomes, pain relief, strength and endurance, and higher rate of return to preinjury level of sport than nonoperative treatment. Given the uniformly poor outcomes from nonoperative treatment for these injuries, we recommend surgical treatment for acute complete proximal hamstring ruptures in active patients, especially the elite athlete.

Klingele and Sallay[4] reported on a series of 11 patients who underwent surgical treatment for complete proximal hamstring tendon ruptures. Ten of 11 patients were

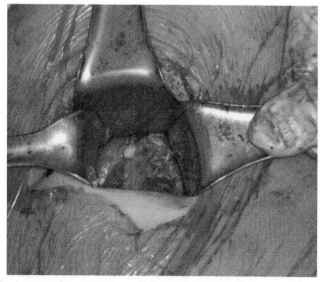

Fig. 5. The final repair after sutures are tied down over the proximal hamstring tendon.

Box 1
Postoperative rehabilitation protocol after proximal hamstring tendon repair

Rehabilitation Protocol Following Acute Proximal Hamstring Repair[3,26]

GENERAL	**Weight Bearing** 0–2 weeks: Toe-touch weight bearing (10% of weight) 2–4 weeks: 25% weight bearing 4–6 weeks: 50% weight bearing 6+ weeks: weight bearing as tolerated **Hip Brace** (set at neutral abduction) Worn at all times for the first 6 weeks after surgery 0–2 weeks = 0–30 degrees 2–4 weeks = 0–45 degrees 4–6 weeks = 0–60 degrees 6 weeks = discontinue brace
WEEK 0	Ankle pumps Supine quadriceps sets–only bring heel 6 inches off the ground (no more than brace will allow)
WEEK 2	Begin formal physical therapy with a physical therapist Passive, **GENTLE**, pain-free range of motion of the hip and knee (avoid concomitant hip flexion and knee extension) Begin submaximal isometric hip abduction and adduction Posterior thigh soft tissue and patella mobilizations
WEEK 4	Begin active quad sets out of brace–limit flexion of hip to what patient can do without any hamstring discomfort/pulling Continue passive only hip extension (no active hamstring exercises) Begin lumbopelvic stabilization exercises Advance calf stretching and ankle strengthening with hip in full extension
WEEK 6	Normal gait training Progress passive and active ranges of motion Begin active hamstring exercises: hamstring curls, prone planks with hip extension, etc. (only against gravity; no added weight) Begin isotonic exercises within a limited range of motion (avoiding the terminal ranges of motion) Begin core pelvic strength training and closed-chain exercises Prone quad strengthening Single and double limb balance and proprioception exercises Begin aquatherapy (if incision well healed)
MONTH 2	Slowly add resistance to hamstring exercises as tolerated (progress isotonic strength training) Advance dynamic training (mini-squats, mini-lunges, resisted side-stepping, grape-vines, etc.) Begin stationary bike without resistance when patient has 90 degrees of hip flexion Hydroworx pool allowed for early return to jogging
MONTH 3	Begin light jogging Continue strengthening hamstrings/quads/gluts
MONTH 4–5	May advance jogging as tolerated (no aggressive acceleration) Incorporate sport-specific activities (agility progression) Begin plyometric exercises
MONTH 6–9	Return to unrestricted activity/sports once patient has returned to full contra-lateral leg strength and endurance levels

satisfied with the result, and 7 of 9 athletically active patients were able to return to sport an average of 6 months (range, 3 to 10) after surgery. In cases of complete avulsion with hamstring retraction, a delay in surgical repair renders the repair more technically challenging and may increase the likelihood of sciatic nerve involvement.[5]

Patients may also be deemed to be surgical candidates if they suffer from what is now referred to as "hamstring syndrome." Patients who suffer from this syndrome usually have a history of chronic hamstring strains.[12] These patients commonly complain of pain in the area of the ischial tuberosity with radiation down the posterior thigh. Chronic tendinopathy or chronic ruptures in the proximal hamstring can cause scar tissue to involve the sciatic nerve. As a result, contraction of the hamstring causes traction on the nerve and subsequent symptoms. Young and van Riet[27] showed good results in a study of 43 patients who underwent a surgical release for this specific diagnosis.

Preferred Surgical Technique

Our preferred surgical technique is one that has been proposed by Cohen and Bradley.[3] The patient is positioned prone on the operating table, and a transverse incision is made in the gluteal crease, centered over the ischial tuberosity. The gluteus maximus is retracted superiorly, and the fascia of the hamstring tendons is incised longitudinally. The sciatic nerve is identified along the lateral border and protected throughout the case. The proximal hamstring tendon stump is debrided and tagged with suture (**Fig. 3**). Attention is then turned to removing all of the scar tissue from the ischial tuberosity to facilitate healing. Five bioabsorbable suture anchors are then drilled and inserted in an "X" configuration on the posterolateral aspect of the ischial tuberosity (**Fig. 4**). The sutures from the anchors are passed through the tendon and tied down using a horizontal mattress configuration (**Fig. 5**). Postoperatively, weight bearing is advanced from 10 pounds on the operative extremity to weight bearing as tolerated over 6 weeks. Patients are given a hip orthosis in neutral abduction, limiting hip flexion to 30° and gradually increasing it over 6 weeks to decrease stress on the repair (knee range of motion is unlimited in the brace). Gentle hip range of motion is begun under close supervision at week 2 and slowly advanced over the following 4 to 6 weeks. Strengthening exercises are advanced after 3 months postoperatively. Full return to activity is allowed 6 to 9 months after surgery. Our full postoperative rehabilitation protocol is attached as **Box 1**.

SUMMARY

Hamstring injuries continue to be very common for both elite and amateur athletes. Given their high recurrence rate, the ability to treat these injuries effectively is critical to helping athletes return to their previous level of activity without putting them at risk for future injury. Most hamstring strains can be treated with initial pain control and a course of rehabilitation focused on a gradual return to activity. However, an exact, evidence-based rehabilitation protocol has yet to be studied. Although surgery is rare and reserved for complete hamstring ruptures, results show high patient satisfaction and ability to return to play.

REFERENCES

1. Orchard J, Best TM, Verrall GM. Return to play following muscle strains. Clin J Sport Med 2005;15:436–41.
2. Clanton TO, Coupe KJ. Hamstring strains in athletes: diagnosis and treatment. J Am Acad Orthop Surg 1998;6:237–48.

3. Cohen SB, Bradley J. Acute proximal hamstring rupture. J Am Acad Orthop Surg 2007;15:350–5.
4. Klingele KE, Sallay PI. Surgical repair of complete proximal hamstring tendon rupture. Am J Sports Med 2002;30(5):742–7.
5. Wood DG, Packham I, Trikha SP, et al. Avulsion of the proximal hamstring origin. Bone Joint Surg Am 2008;90(11):2365–74.
6. Harris JD, Griesser MJ. Treatment of proximal hamstring ruptures: a systematic review. Int J Sports Med 2011;32(7):490–5.
7. Beltran L, Ghazikhanian V, Padron M, et al. The proximal hamstring muscle-tendon-bone unit: a review of the normal anatomy, biomechanics, and pathophysiology. Eur J Radiol 2011. [Epub ahead of print].
8. Garrett WE Jr, Best TM. Anatomy, physiology, and mechanics of skeletal muscle. In: Simon SR, editor. Orthopaedic basic science. Rosemont, Ill: American Academy of Orthopaedic Surgeons; 1994. p. 89–125.
9. Verrall G, Slavotinek J. Clinical risk factors for hamstring muscle strain injury: a prospective study with correlation of injury by magnetic resonance imaging. Br J Sports Med 2001;335(6):435–9.
10. Foreman TK, Addy T, Baker S, et al. Prospective studies into the causation of hamstring injuries in sport: a systematic review. Physical Therapy in Sport 2006;7(2): 101–9.
11. Gabbe B, Finch C, Bennell KL, et al. Risk factors for hamstring injuries in community level Australian football. Br J Sports Med 2005;39(2):106–10.
12. Engebretsen A, Myklebust I, Holme I, et al. Intrinsic risk factors for hamstring injuries among male soccer players: a prospective cohort study. Am J Sports Med 2010;38(6):1147–53.
13. Puranen J, Orava S. The hamstring syndrome: a new diagnosis of gluteal sciatic pain. Am J Sports Med 1988;16(5):517–21.
14. Heiderscheit BC, Sherry MA, Silder A, et al. Hamstring strain injuries: recommendations for diagnosis, rehabilitation, and injury prevention. Cochrane Database Syst Rev 2007;1:CD004575.
15. Petersen J, Holmich P. Evidence based prevention of hamstring injuries in sport. J Orthop Sports Phys Ther 2010;40(2):67–81.
16. Worrell TW. Factors associated with hamstring injuries. An approach to treatment and preventative measures. Br J Sports Med 2011. [Epub ahead of print].
17. Mendiguchia J, Alentorn-Geli E, Brughelli M. Hamstring strain injuries: are we heading in the right direction? N Am J Sports Phys Ther 2008;3(2):67–81.
18. Hibbert O, Cheong K, Grant A, et al. A systematic review of the effectiveness of eccentric strengthening in the prevention of hamstring muscle strains in otherwise healthy individuals. Int J Sports Med 2011;32(7):490–5.
19. Mason DL, Dickesn V, Vail A. Rehabilitation for hamstring injuries. Sports Med 1994;17(5):338–45.
20. Garrett WE Jr, Nikolaou PK, Ribbeck BM, et al. The effect of muscle architecture on the biomechanical failure properties of skeletal muscle under passive extension. Am J Sports Med 1988;16:7–12.
21. Goldman EF, Jones DE. Interventions for preventing hamstring injuries: a systematic review. Physiotherapy 2011;97(2):91–9.
22. Levine WN, Bergfeld JA. Intramuscular corticosteroid injection for hamstring injuries. A 13-year experience in the National Football League. Am J Sports Med 2000;28(3): 297–30.

23. Taylor DW, Petrera M, Hendry M, et al. A systematic review of the use of platelet-rich plasma in sports medicine as a new treatment for tendon and ligament injuries. Clin J Sport Med 2011;21(4):344–52.

24. Malliaropoulos N, Isinkaye T, Tsitas K, et al. Reinjury after acute posterior thigh muscle injuries in elite track and field athletes. Br J Sports Med 2005;39(6):319–23.

25. Cohen SB, Towers J, Zoga A, et al. Hamstring injuries in professional football players: MRI correlation with return to play. Sports Health: a multidisciplinary approach 2011. [Epub ahead of print].

26. Kirkland A, Garrison JC, Singleton SB, et al. Surgical and therapeutic management of a complete proximal hamstring avulsion after failed conservative approach. J Orthop Sports Phys Ther 2008;38:754–60.

27. Young I, van Riet R, Bell SN. Surgical release for proximal hamstring syndrome. Am J Sports Med. 2008;36(12):2372–8.

Medial Tibial Stress Syndrome

Noam Reshef, MD[a], David R. Guelich, MD[b],*

KEYWORDS

- Medial tibial stress syndrome • Stress • Reaction • Tibia
- Shin

INTRODUCTION

The first description of medial tibial stress syndrome (MTSS) was in 1958. Devas[1] published the first study and described signs and symptoms of what he termed *stress fracture at the tibia* or *shin soreness*. Other terms like *medial tibial syndrome,*[2] *tibial stress syndrome,*[3] *shin splint syndrome,*[4] and *medial tibial stress syndrome*[5] have followed. Numerous definitions for this condition have been described by experienced sports clinicians, highlighting the vague understanding of this condition. Yates and White[6] most accurately described MTSS as "pain along the posteromedial border of the tibia that occurs during exercise, excluding pain from ischemic origin or signs of stress fracture." The purpose of this review is to summarize the known data about MTSS and to give a formal definition and treatment algorithm, allowing for timely diagnosis and treatment.

RELATED PATHOANATOMY AND PATHOPHYSIOLOGY

MTSS is broadly defined as painful symptoms on the medial aspect of the tibia, often located at the middle or distal portion. There is disagreement about the etiology of MTSS. Numerous theories relating functional anatomy and pathologic biomechanics are the foundation for the development of MTSS. Several cadaveric studies evaluate the relationship between the exact location of the pain and the associated anatomical structures. The traction theory was first published by Devas in 1958,[1] stating that traction to the periosteum can be caused by any strong calf muscle. Namely, the muscle causes tension of the periosteum causing inflammation and eventual bone production. Michael and Holder[7] performed dissection on 14 cadaveric specimens. They concluded the fibers of the soleus muscle insert 4 inches proximal to the medial malleolus. The pain is formed from a fascial covering over the deep compartment of

The authors have nothing to disclose.

[a] Center for Athletic Medicine, 830 West Diversey Pkwy, Chicago, IL 60614, USA
[b] Chicago Orthopedics & Sports Medicine, 3000 North Halsted Avenue, Suite 525, Chicago, IL 60657, USA
* Corresponding author.
E-mail address: drguelich@chiorthosports.com

Clin Sports Med 31 (2012) 273–290
doi:10.1016/j.csm.2011.09.008
0278-5919/12/$ – see front matter © 2012 Elsevier Inc. All rights reserved.

sportsmed.theclinics.com

the leg. Saxena and colleagues[8] believed the tibialis posterior (TP) muscle was the cause for MTSS. By dissecting 10 cadavers, they identified the muscle origin 7.7 cm proximal to medial malleolus and the intersection of the TP and the flexor hallucis longus (FHL) 8.2 cm proximal to the medial malleolus. This intersection point is the source of pain in MTSS and is associated with FHL flexion. Both these studies suggest a traction theory as the pathologic condition.

Beck and Osternig[9] concluded that if a traction etiology was implicated in MTSS, the soleus and the FHL (not the TP) are involved. They dissected 50 legs and found no fibers of the TP muscle on the distal half of the posteromedial border of the tibia. In the upper half of the distal tibia, fibers of the soleus muscle and FHL muscle were abundant on the medial border. Few muscle fibers of the soleus muscle or any other muscle were found at the distal part of the tibia, where MTSS complaints are commonly felt. Garth and Miller[10] suggested that the flexor digitorum longus (FDL) is the cause of MTSS. They evaluated 17 runners with suspected MTSS and noted pain associated with flexion of the metatarsophalangeal joints and a relative weakness of the FHL muscle. They also suggested that MTSS may be associated with mild claw toe deformity. Recently, Bouche and Johnson[11] added support to this theory. Using 3 cadaveric specimens, they applied tension to the tibial periosteum through the soleus, TP, and the FDL muscles. As tension was increased, strain in the tibial fascia and periosteum increased in a linear manner.

Another explanation for the etiology of MTSS is the ability of the calf muscles to cause repeated bending or bowing of the tibia, thereby causing a stress reaction and periosteal reaction.[12] This theory was originally described by Devas[1] and Beck[13] as a possible explanation of posterior calf pain. Several studies found that repeated bending of the tibia causes adaptive reaction of bone, predominantly where bending forces are greatest.[14,15] This is located at the narrowest part of the diaphysis of the tibia, between the middle and the distal third.[16] As described by Wolff's law, repeated loads applied to bone initiate a cascade of signal transduction, detected by the cellular components of bone.[17,18] This response will repair microdamage to a certain threshold. Repetitive load or stress may cause the microdamage to rise above a threshold that escapes repair.[18]

To study the biomechanical properties of the tibia in stress fractures and MTSS, Franklyn and colleagues[19] looked at a cohort of military recruits (men and women) suffering from stress fractures and MTSS. The authors compared them with 2 gender-mixed control groups: aerobically active and sedentary. Using tibial scout radiographs and cross-sectional computed tomography, the aerobic control group had larger cortical cross-sectional area than the inactive subjects in men. Similarly, MTSS and tibial stress fractures had a smaller cortical area than aerobic controls. They calculated that aerobic controls were better adapted to axial loading, torsion, and bending rigidity than subjects with MTSS and tibial stress fractures. They also showed that the MTSS group had lower cross-sectional cortical area compared with aerobic controls in both men and women. This suggests that MTSS is not only a soft tissue problem but may involve the adaption of the distal tibial cortex to repetitive stress.

Studies have also suggested that lower muscle strength has a negative influence on the bone adaptation process. This pathologic condition develops when weak leg muscles cannot oppose the bending forces on the tibia, resulting in greater strain on the tibial cortex.[20,21] Other investigators have suggested a theory in which the adaptation of traction and bony overload is challenged by the traction of the soleus and flexor hallucis longus muscles on the periosteum.[13]

Histologic analysis is also inconclusive. It is thought that tension applied on the periosteum will result in an inflammatory reaction and could explain the pain. Two studies showed a mild inflammatory response. Michael and Holder[7] found inflammation and vasculitis on biopsy of the fascia in 3 patients. Mubarak and coworkers[5] found microscopic inflammation and vasculitis of the periosteum in 2 patients. Other studies with larger cohorts did not find inflammatory changes in the periosteum. Johnell and colleagues[22] found inflammatory tissue in the crural fascia in 13 of 33 legs of athletes who underwent fasciotomy due to exercise-induced pain over the medial edge of the tibia after exercise that failed to respond to conservative treatment. Bhatt and coworkers[23] found plasma cell infiltration surrounding wide lymphatics in the periosteum, along with a thickened periosteum and increased osteoblast activity. They also found fewer osteocytes compared with that of normal bone, although this finding failed to achieve statistical significance. One of the biopsies of Johnell and coworkers[22] noted similar findings. The level of activity and the type of the athletes were not reported.

Magnusson and colleagues[24] found low regional tibial bone density in athletes with MTSS compared with healthy athletes. Dual-energy x-ray absorptiometry showed decreased bone density in the mid to distal tibia (23% ± 8%; mean ± SD) in patients with MTSS. Bone density returned to normal values when the athletes had recovered after a mean of 5.7 years (range, 4–8 years).[25]

It appears that the combination of traction on the periosteum by the calf muscles and repetitive bending loads across the tibia are the main causes of MTSS. These conditions interact, creating a pathologic environment that the body cannot heal. Inflammatory response of the periosteum is a good explanation for the acute stage, whereas degeneration, as demonstrated in biopsies, involves the chronic stage. Bone remodeling is the result of an anabolic periosteal reaction. Although there are histologic and environmental similarities to stress fractures, no study supports progression of MTSS to a stress fracture.

RISK FACTORS

A number of studies address the intrinsic and extrinsic risk factors for MTSS. Intrinsic factors include foot posture, alignment, and ankle flexibility and strength. Foot pronation is often considered a risk factor for MTSS. Yet, the definition of pronation varies. Yates and White,[6] in a study of military recruits, identified the group who suffered from MTSS had a more pronated foot type (P = .002). They evaluated pronation by using the Foot Pronation Index (**Fig. 1**).[26,27] This index is an observational test that determines the position of the foot (pronated, supinated, or neutral) based on 8 parameters. These parameters distinguish frontal, sagittal, and transverse plane positions. Gehlsen and Seger[28] measured the angle between the calcaneus and the midline of the leg during running. They found that angular displacement was significantly greater in the MTSS group compared with the non-MTSS group ($P<.01$). Viitasalo and Kvist[29] found that the angle between the lower leg and calcaneus at heel strike was higher for the symptomatic group ($P<.01$).

The navicular drop test has also been referenced. The navicular drop test is the difference in distance between the lower border of the loaded and unloaded navicular bone and the ground (**Fig. 2**).[30,31] The test is considered an indicator of midfoot pronation. The navicular prominence is also 1 of 8 parameters in the Foot Posture Index.[26,27] Navicular drop test was measured by Bennett et al[30] in 125 high school runners. The mean drop distance in runners with complaints of MTSS was 6.8 mm, compared with 3.7 mm in the asymptomatic group (P = .003). Bandholm et al[32] in a case-control study involving symptomatic athletes showed a significant increase in MTSS symptoms associated with higher navicular drop tests (MTSS group, 7.7; control group, 5.0; P = .046). On the other hand, 2 other prospective studies did not

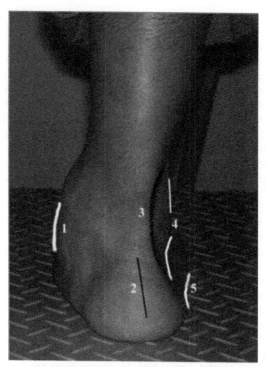

Fig. 1. Posterior view of a pronated foot as defined by the foot posture index. (*1*) Talar navicular prominence; (*2*) calcaneal frontal plane position; (*3*) Helbing's sign; (*4*) inferior and superior lateral malleolar curves; (*5*) congruence of the lateral border. (*From* Yates B, White S. The incidence and risk factors in the development of medial tibial stress syndrome among naval recruits. Am J Sports Med 2004;32(3):772–80; with permission.)

find an increased navicular drop distance in MTSS compared with that in asymptomatic runners.[31,33]

Another way to evaluate foot position is the standing foot angle, which measures the angle between the medial malleolus, navicular prominence, and first metatarsal head. A study by Sommer and Vallentyne[34] found that a standing foot angle less than 140° was predictive of MTSS ($P < .0001$) with a sensitivity and specificity of 71.3% and 69.5% respectively. They also found that subjects with MTSS had higher hindfoot and forefoot varus compared with control subjects ($P = .017$).

Gait analysis has gained popularity, allowing for dynamic evaluation of foot position during walking and running. Bandholm and coworkers[32] evaluated foot properties of recreational athletes with MTSS compared with healthy controls using 3-dimensional gait analysis. The group with MTSS showed increased medial longitudinal-arch deformation (5.9°) during quiet standing compared with controls (5.0° and 3.5°, $P = .05$). Subjects with medial tibial stress syndrome also showed significantly larger medial longitudinal-arch deformation (8.8°) during gait compared with controls (7.1°, $P = .015$). In the study by Tweed and colleagues,[35] 28 athletes were videotaped during running with and without shoes. Three of the variables tested during running were significantly different between the groups, including early heel rise ($P = .003$), abduction of the forefoot ($P = .003$) and a propulsive gait ($P < .001$).

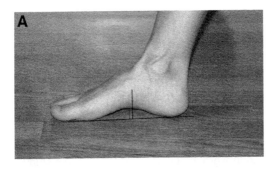

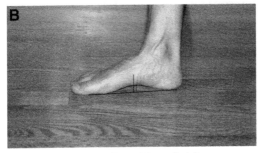

Fig. 2. Navicular drop test. (*A*) Unloaded foot. (*B*) Loaded foot.

Viitasalo and Kvist[29] investigated passive ankle inversion and eversion in a case-control study among male athletes. They found increased passive inversion (19.5°) and eversion (10.7°) in the ankle to be an intrinsic risk factor ($P<.05$). Bennett and colleagues[30] and Burne and coworkers[36] compared male and female groups of healthy individuals and those with MTSS for reduced ankle dorsiflexion. Ankle dorsiflexion for symptomatic men and women was 32° and 29°, respectively, and similar to that in the control group ($P>.05$). Therefore, ankle dorsiflexion was not identified as an intrinsic risk factor for MTSS. Increased plantarflexion range of motion[33] and increased plantarflexion strength[28] were found to be statistically significant risk factors for MTSS.

Burne and coworkers[36] conducted a prospective study looking at risk factors for developing MTSS in Australian military recruits. They found that greater internal and external hip rotation was a risk factor. The amount of internal and external hip range of motion among patients was 8° to 12° increased over asymptomatic controls. They also found that the lean calf girth was 10 to 15 mm less among symptomatic cadets compared with asymptomatic cadets. This finding was only significant among men ($P<.04$). Madeley and coworkers[37] in a case-control study, found a significant difference in the number of heel raises that could be performed. Patients suffering from MTSS did 23 repetitions per minute compared with 33 in the controls ($P<.001$). This finding suggests muscular endurance is also a factor in MTSS.

In a prospective study evaluating risk factors for MTSS in runners,[31] the authors found that a higher body mass index (>20) is an intrinsic risk factor in cross-country runners. Female sex is also considered an intrinsic risk factor. Yates and White,[6] in a prospective study of naval recruits in Australia, showed MTSS incidence of 52.9% in women compared with 28.2% in men (relative risk [RR], 2.03). Another prospective study involving Australian Defense Force Academy recruits[36] also showed female sex to be a risk factor (MTSS incidence: women, 30.6%; men, 9.8%; overall risk [OR], 3.1). A third study evaluating the incidence of MTSS in a group of high school cross-country runners showed that females had 5.46 times more MTSS than males (19.1% in females and 3.5% in males, $P<.003$).[30]

Several studies have looked at extrinsic factors in the development of MTSS. In a retrospective, case-control study on running injuries by Tounton and colleagues[38] it was found that an activity history of less than 8.5 years was an extrinsic risk factor (OR, 3.5 in men, 2.5 in women). The results were confirmed in a prospective study by Hubbard and coworkers[33] showing that athletes with MTSS had been running fewer years (5.3) than the control group (8.8; $P = .002$). The same study found athletes with a previous history of MTSS had higher risk of MTSS development than those who did not have MTSS in the past ($P = .0001$).

Multiple risk factors are considered significant in the development of MTSS: female sex, excessive pronation, increased internal and external hip rotation, body mass index greater than 21, small/lean calf girth, previous history of MTSS, and inexperienced runner. Other risk factors, such as increased running intensity, longer running distance, running on different terrains, changes in running shoes or running in old shoes, are mentioned, but no studies support them as risk factors for MTSS.

PATIENT EVALUATION
Signs and Symptoms

The differential diagnosis of exercise-induced leg pain includes medial tibial stress syndrome, tibial stress fracture, exertional compartment syndrome, and popliteal artery entrapment and nerve entrapment.[39] However, history usually eliminates most nerve and vascular conditions, leaving chronic exertional compartment syndrome, stress fracture, and MTSS.

MTSS presents as running-induced leg pain. Commonly, the pain is located along the posteromedial border of the tibia, usually in the middle or distal thirds. Initially, the symptoms are present with early activity and subside with continued exercise, but may persist throughout activity. When the condition deteriorates, the pain is felt even after the activity ends and may be present at rest.[40] In severe cases, the symptoms may appear with little provocation and with simple activities. This presentation is also associated with stress fractures. The clinician must approach these patients with a higher index of suspicion.

Physical Examination

Physical examination of the patient with MTSS focuses on several aspects: accurate location of the symptoms, evaluation of postural risk factors related to MTSS, and elimination of other conditions associated with runners. When performing an examination, pain should be present with palpation of the distal two-thirds of the posteromedial border of the tibia. Mild swelling at the posteromedial border of tibia may also be present.[39,40] Moen and colleagues[41] attempted to determine the sensitivity and specificity of physical examination tests. Symptomatic athletes and a control group of athletes were included. The gold standard in this study was bone scintigraphy. Three tests were examined: diffuse posteromedial pain on palpation, pain on hopping, and pain on percussion. Diffuse posteromedial pain on palpation was the most sensitive finding.

In chronic exertional compartment syndrome, patients usually describe a painful, exercise-related tightness over the anterolateral aspect of the leg. This may be accompanied by mild neurologic symptoms. The pain does not appear at rest, but usually increases during activity and resolves quickly when the physical effort is ceased. No tenderness is noted on direct palpation. Diagnosis is clinical and is confirmed using intracompartmental pressure measurements before exercise and 1 minute and 2 minutes after exercise.[39] Past theories related MTSS to elevated intracompartmental pressure of the posterior compartment. Several authors investigated this theory. Puranen and Alavaikko[42] measured the pressure in the medial compartment in 22 athletes with medial-sided leg pain. They found that on exercise, the pressure was substantially higher in the symptomatic patients than in the control group; after fasciotomy, the pressure returned to normal limits. Other studies failed to reproduce the same results. One study evaluated track runners clinically diagnosed with MTSS but showed no elevation of compartmental pressures.[5] Other studies found a lower intracompartmental pressure in a group with MTSS compared with the pressure found in a group with chronic exertional compartment syndrome.[43,44]

Differentiating MTSS and stress fracture is more challenging. Pain characteristics may be similar. In patients with stress fractures, tenderness is more localized[45] and usually located in the middle anterior one-third of the tibia.[46] X-rays are usually normal in the first few weeks, followed by formation of callus, confirming the exact location of the stress fracture.[47] Diagnosis is usually made or confirmed by bone scintigraphy or magnetic resonance imaging (MRI).[48] Stress fractures originating in the posterior distal third of the tibia are unusual.

Imaging Studies

Numerous studies have been published concerning diagnostic imaging and MTSS. The necessity of imaging studies in the setting of a thorough history and examination has been questioned[49–52] but are necessary when concern regarding stress fracture is significant. Radiographs are usually the first step in the orthopedic imaging evaluation. Edwards and colleagues[40] mentioned the use of x-ray as a preliminary study but mainly to rule out other causes of leg pain. In one study, Batt and colleagues[53] showed periosteal reaction on the posteromedial aspect of the tibia in 4 of 46 patients with MTSS. Two other studies described callus formation, but the accurate diagnosis of MTSS was not clear.[5,7]

Using bone scintigraphy for the diagnosis of MTSS was first described by Holder and Michael.[50] They evaluated patients with clinically diagnosed MTSS using triple-phase bone scintigraphy (angiogram, blood pool images, and delayed images). The first 2 phases showed no absorption. On the delayed phase, a longitudinal lesion at the posterior aspect of the tibia involving one third of the tibia was noted (**Fig. 3**). The authors suggested that MTSS is a condition that irritates the periosteum, causing activation of osteoblasts. Similar conclusions were noted by other authors.[54,55] The sensitivity of bone scintigraphy in diagnosing MTSS is 74% to 84%.[49,53] Zwas and colleagues[56] and Matin[57] published staging criteria for bone scintigraphic findings related mainly to stress fractures. These scales attempted to differentiate between stress fractures and MTSS, although it was shown to be difficult and inaccurate.[53,54] Overdiagnosis and false-positive findings of bone scintigraphy have been documented. Batt and coworkers[53] noted 80% of asymptomatic athletes undergoind bone scintigraphy demonstrated pathologic findings. False-positive bone scan result was found in several studies,[50,54] calling into question the routine use of bone scintigraphy in evaluating MTSS.

MRI is gaining popularity in cases of suspected MTSS, mainly because periosteal and bony edema are easily seen (**Fig. 4**).[52] Batt and colleagues[53]and Gaeta and colleagues[49] showed sensitivity of 78% to 89% and specificity of 33% and 100%,

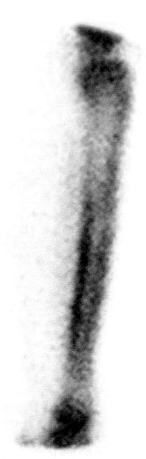

Fig. 3. Medial view of the tibia on isotope bone Scintigraphy: tubular pattern characteristic of medial tibial syndrome. (*From* Bhatt R, Lauder I, Finlay DB, et al. Correlation of bone scintigraphy and histological findings in medial tibial syndrome. Br J Sports Med 2000;34(1): 49–53; with permission.)

respectively. Fredericson and colleagues[58] developed a grading system for stress reaction in runners based on clinical findings, bone scan, and MRI. According to his study, patients with grade 1 or 2 (grade 1, positive short tau inversion recovery [STIR] image;, grade 2, positive STIR and positive T2-weighted image) had posteromedial tenderness upon physical examination; whereas patients with grade 3 to 4 had local tenderness over the medial tibial diaphysis. The authors did not find a correlation between bone scintigraphy and MRI findings in MTSS patients. In another study, Batt and coworkers[53] did find a positive correlation.

Arendt and Griffiths[59] modified Fredericson's grading system. Using Fredericson's classification, they defined grade 1 and 2 as "low grade stress fracture" or "stress reaction phenomenon" which correlates with MTSS and is a different entity. Grades 3 and 4 are considered "high grade stress fracture" or "classic stress fracture" and are a different entity. They used their system to determine return to play time of patients with MTSS. Grade 1 patients returned to play in 4 weeks and grade 2 returned to play in 6 weeks, whereas classic stress fractures are treated more cautiously with

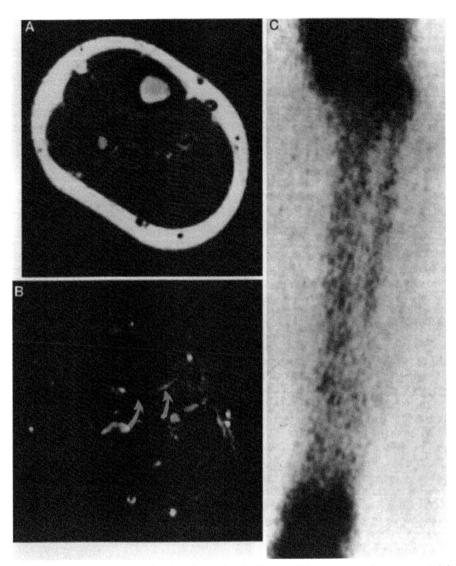

Fig. 4. Grade 1 MRI findings in right lower leg in 19-year-old woman varsity runner. Axial T1-weighted MR image (*A*) shows no detectable abnormality, but the T2-weighted image (*B*) shows mild periosteal edema along the posteromedial aspect of the tibial cortex (*curved arrows*), with normal bone marrow signal. Bone scintigraphy (*C*) shows mild diffuse increase in activity, which was not present in the contralateral lower extremity Grade. (*Adapted from* Fredericson M, Bergman AG, Hoffman KL, et al. Tibial stress reaction in runners. Correlation of clinical symptoms and scintigraphy with a new magnetic resonance imaging grading system. Am J Sports Med 1995;23(4):472–8; with permission.)

prolonged rest. Aoki and coworkers[51] showed a linear, abnormally high signal in the posteromedial border of the tibia in the early stages of the syndrome. Five patients had follow-up MRI 4 weeks later and showed no progression to a stress fracture. Anderson and colleagues[52] showed that in chronic cases of MTSS (over 46 months of symptoms), MRI was normal in 7 of 19 patients. False-positive MRI findings were found in 21 runners who ran 80 to 100 km per week for 8 weeks. Forty-three percent of those runners showed abnormal findings related to tibial stress reaction despite all the runners being asymptomatic.[60]

High-resolution computerized tomography is another modality that was evaluated for its accuracy in MTSS. Gaeta and colleagues[49,61] documented posteromedial cortical osteopenia in patient with MTSS, noting a sensitivity of 42% and specificity of 100%. Another study found the case group (11 runners with unilateral or bilateral MTSS) had cortical osteopenia, whereas 8 of 48 asymptomatic legs had cortical osteopenia. Sensitivity, specificity, positive predictive value, negative predictive value, and accuracy of computed tomography in diagnosing medial tibial stress syndrome were 100%, 88.2%, 63.6%, 100%, and 90.2%, respectively.

MTSS is a clinical diagnosis, and radiographic imaging should only be utilized when the diagnosis is in question. Routine plain radiographs are of little benefit when the diagnosis of MTSS is clear on history and physical examination. MRI is the most accurate study when the patient is symptomatic and may help differentiate between MTSS and advanced stress fracture. Other modalities may be used accordingly if the diagnosis remains in question. Data regarding the accuracy and effectiveness of different imaging modalities is summarized in **Table 1**. Differentiating between MTSS and an early stress fracture is still a radiographic challenge.

TREATMENT

Conservative treatment consists of the common modalities: rest, ice, compression, and elevation. Bracing, physical therapy, and stretching are also utilized. Andrish and coworkers[62] conducted a randomized, controlled study on 97 marine recruits who had MTSS. The patients were divided to 5 groups: group 1, no running, ice pack on the painful area 3 times daily; group 2, 4 times daily was added to the treatment regime for 1 week; group 3, 100 mg phenylbutazone 4 times daily was added for 1 week; group 4, calf muscle stretching 3 times a day for 3 minutes; group 5, a plaster walking cast was applied for 1 week. Duration of pain before treatment was 1 to 14 days, and the marines were considered recovered if no pain or tenderness remained when 500 meters of running was completed. The time to recovery for each group was: group 1, 6.4 days; group 2, 9.4 days, group 3, 7.5 days; group 4, 8.8 days; and group 5, 10.8 days. The mean time to recovery was 8.6 days. No significant difference was found between the treatment groups.

Another study by Nissen and colleagues[63] evaluated low-energy laser treatment. It was designed as double blind study and also involved military cadets. The cadets were divided into 2 groups. One group (26 patients) was treated with low energy laser device, and the second group was treated with placebo device. Each of the 2 groups received a maximum of 6 treatments per patient, and Visual Analog Score was recorded before each treatment. The ability to return to full duty was evaluated by a physician after 14 days or a maximum of 6 treatments and was based on physical examination and patient history. Eighteen of 23 patients (78%) of the placebo group and 19 of 26 (73%) in the treatment group were able to return to full duty after 14 days. No statistical significance was found in VAS scores.

Loudon and Dolphino[64] evaluated a group of runners with MTSS, treated with calf stretching and off-the-shelf basic orthoses. Fifteen of the 23 patients showed 50% reduction of their symptoms after 3 weeks of intervention. They concluded that orthoses may be used as a part of the treatment in MTSS, but should be combined with other methods. Moen and colleagues[65], in a randomized trial, examined the effectiveness of pneumatic leg brace in the treatment of MTSS in military recruits and found no additional value. Low Energy Extracorporal shock wave therapy (ESWT) was evaluated by Rompe and coworkers[66] in a case control study. Ninety-four patients with recalcitrant MTSS were divided into 2 groups. The treatment group (47 patients) were treated with home training program and received repetitive low-energy radial Shock Wave Treatment. The control group was treated with home training program only. Degree of recovery was measured on a 6-point Likert scale (subjects with a rating of completely recovered or much improved were rated as treatment success). One month, 4 months, and 15 months from onset of symptoms, success rates for the control and treatment groups according to the Likert scale were 13% and 30% ($P<.001$), 30% and 64% ($P<.001$), and 37% and 76% ($P<.001$), respectively. At 15 months from baseline, 40 of the 47 subjects in the treatment group had been able to return to their preferred sport at their pre-injury level, as had 22 of the 47 control subjects. They concluded that low energy ESWT is a good treatment for recalcitrant MTSS. Moen and colleagues[67], in a prospective observational control trial, found that runners treated with a combined graded running program and ESWT returned to normal activity faster than runners that were treated with graded running program alone ($P = .008$). Other studies have been published, showing the effectiveness of several treatment modalities like acupuncture[68] but these article have limited strength.

Surgical treatment is rarely indicated in MTS but has been evaluated in several studies. Different surgical approaches were described including fasciotomy along the posteromedial border of the tibia both under both general and local anesthesia.[69–71] Other authors added a removal of a periosteal strip form the posteromedial border, reducing the traction over the periosteum.[72,73] These studies report generally positive outcomes with good to excellent results in 69% to 92%.[71,72] Return to pre-injury levels was generally less favorable, varying between 31% and 93%.[72]

PREVENTION

Numerous approaches for prevention of MTSS have been published. The central premise is that MTSS is an overuse injury, "too much, too fast, too soon." Most studies regarding prevention are done with military recruits. In 1974, Andrish and colleagues[62] conducted a study on 2777 military recruits who were divided randomly into 5 groups. Group 1 served as a control group and performed the normal training regimen. The other 4 groups were enrolled in a similar training regimen but had a preventative intervention added. One group wore heel pads in their shoes. Another performed heel-cord stretching exercises 3 times daily for 3 minutes. A third group performed stretching exercises and wore a heel pad. The last group entered a gradual running program 2 weeks before the start of the training schedule and equaled the rest of the groups during the third week of training. No significant difference was found between the different groups in incidence of MTSS. Incidence rates were, consecutively, 3.0% in the control group, 4.4% in the heel pad group, 4.0% in the stretching group, 3.0% in the heel pad plus stretching group, and 6.0% in the group with a graduated running program. Another randomized, controlled study by Schwellnus and colleagues[74] included 1538 soldiers, of whom 237 were randomly assigned to an intervention group. They performed 9 weeks of training. The control group wore standard insoles, and the intervention group wore neoprene insoles. After 9 weeks of training, 20.4% of the control group had MTSS compared with 12.8% in the intervention group. This was a significant difference, although the definition of MTSS was not clear. Another study[75] evaluated the addition of calcium as a method of preventing MTSS with no statistical significance. Larsen and colleagues[76] evaluated the influence of custom-made shoe orthoses in back and lower extremity pain. They

Table 1
Imaging studies for MTSS - data collection

Study	Number of	TPBS				CT				MRI				Comments
		Sensitivity	Specificity	PPV	NPV	Sensitivity	Specificity	PPV	NPV	Sensitivity	Specificity	PPV	NPV	
Mubarak et al[5]	12	—	—	—	—	Not enough data to determine				—	—	—	—	—
Michael & Holder[7]	N/A	—	—	—	—	Not enough data to determine				—	—	—	—	—
Edwards et al[40]	N/A	—	—	—	—	Not enough data to determine				—	—	—	—	—
Gaeta et al[49]	N/A	74	NC	NC	NC	42	100	100	26	88	100	100	62	—
Holder & Michael[50]	10	90	100	90	90	—	—	—	—	—	—	—	—	—
Aoki et al[51]	14 MTSS, 8 stress tibial fracture	—	—	—	—	—	—	—	—	100	100	—	—	—
Anderson et al[52]	19	—	—	—	—	—	—	—	—	—	—	—	—	Different patterns: normal (n = 7), periosteal fluid only (n = 5), abnormal marrow signal intensity (n = 5), and stress fracture (n = 2).
Batt et al[53]	23 (41 legs)	84	33	—	—	—	—	—	—	79	33	—	—	Assuming TPBS as the "gold-standard," MRI findings demonstrated a sensitivity of 95% and specificity of 67%.

Study							Comments
Chisin et al[54]	27	—	—	—	—	—	—	Lack of good definition of symptom did not allow calculation
Nielsen et al[55]	22 (29 legs)	—	—	—	—	—	—	X-Ray: 45% abnormal. TPBS: 83% abnormal uptake; 17% normal
Zwas et al[56]	235	—	—	—	—	—	—	391 lesions were diagnosed. 40% were a symptomatic. Used as a study to develop classification for stress fractures diagnosis using TPBS
Matin[57]		Not enough data to determine						—
Fredericson et al[58]	14 (18 legs)	—	—	—	—	—	—	All legs had positive finding s in TPBS and MRI. Correlation between TPBS and MRI - 78%
Arendt & Griffiths[59]	26	—	—	—	—	—	—	More severe the lesion on MRI correlates to longer time to return to sport
Bergman et al[60]	21	—	—	—	57	100	—	43% positive findings in 21 asymptomatic runners
Gaeta et al[61]	41	100	88.2	63.6	100	—	—	—

Abbreviations: CT, computed tomography; N/A, not available; NPV, negative predictive value; PPV, positive predictive value; TPBS, triple phase bone scan.

evaluated 146 soldiers who were randomly assigned to receive semirigid custom insoles versus standard insoles. After 3 months of training, MTSS developed in 24 (38%) soldiers with the standard insole, compared with 4 (8%) in the intervention group. This was a significant difference ($P<.005$) although MTSS was not defined. Pope and colleagues[77] evaluated stretching as a preventive method for lower limb injuries. In this study, no effect on the occurrence of MTSS was found between control group and treatment group. A study by Brushoy and colleagues[78] examined the success of a prevention training program during 12 weeks of military training and the incidence of MTSS. Two types of training programs were evaluated on the platoons: leg strength and coordination, and a regular (placebo) training program consisting of strengthening and stretching exercises of the upper body. MTSS was defined as pain on the medial border of the tibia during running, and pain on palpation of the medial tibial border, not localized to one spot. No significant differences were noted between the training groups.

SUMMARY

MTSS is a benign, though painful, condition, and a common problem in the running athlete. It is prevalent among military personnel, runners, and dancers, showing an incidence of 4% to 35%. Common names for this problem include shin splints, soleus syndrome, tibial stress syndrome, and periostitis. The exact cause of this condition is unknown. Previous theories included an inflammatory response of the periosteum or periosteal traction reaction. More recent evidence suggests a painful stress reaction of bone.

The most proven risk factors are hyperpronation of the foot, female sex, and history of previous MTSS. Patient evaluation is based on meticulous history taking and physical examination. Even though the diagnosis remains clinical, imaging studies, such as plain radiographs and bone scans are usually sufficient, although MRI is useful in borderline cases to rule out more significant pathology.

Conservative treatment is almost always successful and includes several options; though none has proven more superior to rest. Prevention programs do not seem to influence the rate of MTSS, though shock-absorbing insoles have reduced MTSS rates in military personnel, and ESWT has shortened the duration of symptoms. Surgery is rarely indicated but has shown some promising results in patients who have not responded to all conservative options.

REFERENCES

1. Devas MB. Stress fractures of the tibia in athletes or shin soreness. J Bone Joint Surg Br 1958;40-B(2):227–39.
2. Clement DB. Tibial stress syndrome in athletes. J Sports Med 1974;2(2):81–5.
3. Puranen J. The medial tibial syndrome: exercise ischaemia in the medial fascial compartment of the leg. J Bone Joint Surg Br 1974;56-B(4):712–5.
4. Slocum DB. The shin splint syndrome. Medical aspects and differential diagnosis. Am J Surg 1967;114(6):875–81.
5. Mubarak SJ, Gould RN, Lee YF, et al. The medial tibial stress syndrome. A cause of shin splints. Am J Sports Med 1982;10(4):201–5.
6. Yates B, White S. The incidence and risk factors in the development of medial tibial stress syndrome among naval recruits. Am J Sports Med 2004;32(3):772–80.
7. Michael RH, Holder LE. The soleus syndrome. A cause of medial tibial stress (shin splints). Am J Sports Med 1985;13(2):87–94.
8. Saxena A, O'Brien T, Bunce D. Anatomic dissection of the tibialis posterior muscle and its correlation to medial tibial stress syndrome. J Foot Surg 1990;29(2):105–8.

9. Beck BR, Osternig LR. Medial tibial stress syndrome. The location of muscles in the leg in relation to symptoms. J Bone Joint Surg Am 1994;76(7):1057–61.
10. Garth WP Jr, Miller ST. Evaluation of claw toe deformity, weakness of the foot intrinsics, and posteromedial shin pain. Am J Sports Med 1989;17(6):821–7.
11. Bouche RT, Johnson CH. Medial tibial stress syndrome (tibial fasciitis): a proposed pathomechanical model involving fascial traction. J Am Podiatr Med Assoc 2007; 97(1):31–6.
12. Goodship AE, Lanyon LE, McFie H. Functional adaptation of bone to increased stress. An experimental study. J Bone Joint Surg Am 1979;61(4):539–46.
13. Beck BR. Tibial stress injuries. An aetiological review for the purposes of guiding management. Sports Med 1998;26(4):265–79.
14. Gross TS, Edwards JL, McLeod KJ, et al. Strain gradients correlate with sites of periosteal bone formation. J Bone Miner Res 1997;12(6):982–8.
15. Judex S, Gross TS, Zernicke RF. Strain gradients correlate with sites of exercise-induced bone-forming surfaces in the adult skeleton. J Bone Miner Res 1997;12(10): 1737–45.
16. Milgrom C, Giladi M, Simkin A, et al. The area moment of inertia of the tibia: a risk factor for stress fractures. J Biomech 1989;22(11-12):1243–8.
17. Frost HM. From Wolff's law to the Utah paradigm: insights about bone physiology and its clinical applications. Anat Rec 2001;262(4):398–419.
18. Frost HM. A 2003 update of bone physiology and Wolff's Law for clinicians. Angle Orthod 2004;74(1):3–15.
19. Franklyn M, Oakes B, Field B, et al. Section modulus is the optimum geometric predictor for stress fractures and medial tibial stress syndrome in both male and female athletes. Am J Sports Med 2008;36(6):1179–89.
20. Milgrom C, Radeva-Petrova DR, Finestone A, et al. The effect of muscle fatigue on in vivo tibial strains. J Biomech 2007;40(4):845–50.
21. Paul IL, Munro MB, Abernethy PJ, et al. Musculo-skeletal shock absorption: relative contribution of bone and soft tissues at various frequencies. J Biomech 1978;11(5): 237–9.
22. Johnell O, Rausing A, Wendeberg B, et al. Morphological bone changes in shin splints. Clin Orthop Relat Res 1982;(167):180–4.
23. Bhatt R, Lauder I, Finlay DB, et al. Correlation of bone scintigraphy and histological findings in medial tibial syndrome. Br J Sports Med 2000;34(1):49–53.
24. Magnusson HI, Westlin NE, Nyqvist F, et al. Abnormally decreased regional bone density in athletes with medial tibial stress syndrome. Am J Sports Med 2001;29(6): 712–5.
25. Magnusson HI, Ahlborg HG, Karlsson C, et al. Low regional tibial bone density in athletes with medial tibial stress syndrome normalizes after recovery from symptoms. Am J Sports Med 2003;31(4):596–600.
26. Redmond AC, Crosbie J, Ouvrier A. Development and validation of a novel rating system for scoring standing foot posture: The Foot Posture Index. Clin Biomech (Bristol, Avon) 2006;21(1):89–98.
27. Keenan AM, Redmond AC, Horton M, et al. The Foot Posture Index: Rasch analysis of a novel, foot-specific outcome measure. Arch Phys Med Rehabil 2007;88(1):88–93.
28. Gehlsen GM, Seger A. Selected measures of angular displacement, strength, and flexibility in subjects with and without shin splints. Res Q Exerc Sport 1980;51(3): 478–85.
29. Viitasalo JT, Kvist M. Some biomechanical aspects of the foot and ankle in athletes with and without shin splints. Am J Sports Med 1983;11(3):125–30.

30. Bennett JE, Reinking MF, Pluemer B, et al. Factors contributing to the development of medial tibial stress syndrome in high school runners. J Orthop Sports Phys Ther 2001; 31(9):504–10.

31. Plisky MS, Rauh MJ, Heiderscheit B, et al. Medial tibial stress syndrome in high school cross-country runners: incidence and risk factors. J Orthop Sports Phys Ther 2007; 37(2):40–7.

32. Bandholm T, Boysen L, Haugaard S, et al. Foot medial longitudinal-arch deformation during quiet standing and gait in subjects with medial tibial stress syndrome. J Foot Ankle Surg 2008;47(2):89–95.

33. Hubbard TJ, Carpenter EM, Cordova ML. Contributing factors to medial tibial stress syndrome: a prospective investigation. Med Sci Sports Exerc 2009; 41(3):490–6.

34. Somme HM, Vallentyne SW. Effect of foot posture on the incidence of medial tibial stress syndrome. Med Sci Sports Exerc 1995;27(6):800–4.

35. Tweed JL, Campbell JA, Avil SJ. Biomechanical risk factors in the development of medial tibial stress syndrome in distance runners. J Am Podiatr Med Assoc 2008; 98(6):436–44.

36. Burne SG, Khan KM, Boudville PB, et al. Risk factors associated with exertional medial tibial pain: a 12 month prospective clinical study. Br J Sports Med 2004;38(4): 441–5.

37. Madeley LT, Munteanu SE, Bonanno DR. Endurance of the ankle joint plantar flexor muscles in athletes with medial tibial stress syndrome: a case-control study. J Sci Med Sport 2007;10(6):356–62.

38. Taunton JE, Ryan MB, Clement DB, et al. A retrospective case-control analysis of 2002 running injuries. Br J Sports Med 2002;36(2):95–101.

39. Edwards PH Jr, Wright ML, Hartman JF. A practical approach for the differential diagnosis of chronic leg pain in the athlete. Am J Sports Med 2005;33(8):1241–9.

40. Kortebein PM, Kaufman KR, Basford JR, et al. Medial tibial stress syndrome. Med Sci Sports Exerc 2000;32(3 Suppl):S27–33.

41. Moen MH, Tol JL, Weir A, et al. Medial tibial stress syndrome: a critical review. Sports Med 2009;39(7):523–46.

42. Puranen J, Alavaikko A. Intracompartmental pressure increase on exertion in patients with chronic compartment syndrome in the leg. J Bone Joint Surg Am 1981;63(8): 1304–9.

43. Wallensten R, Eriksson E. Intramuscular pressures in exercise-induced lower leg pain. Int J Sports Med 1984;5(1):31–5.

44. D'Ambrosia RD, Zelis RF, Chuinard RG, et al. Interstitial pressure measurements in the anterior and posterior compartments in athletes with shin splints. Am J Sports Med 1977;5(3):127–31.

45. Matheson GO, Clement DB, McKenzie DC, et al. Stress fractures in athletes. A study of 320 cases. Am J Sports Med 1987;15(1):46–58.

46. Milgrom C, Giladi M, Stein M, et al. Medial tibial pain. A prospective study of its cause among military recruits. Clin Orthop Relat Res 1986;(213):167–71.

47. Lassus J, Tulikoura I, Konttinen YT, et al. Bone stress injuries of the lower extremity: a review. Acta Orthop Scand 2002;73(3):3568–9.

48. Moran DS, Evans RK, Hadad E. Imaging of lower extremity stress fracture injuries. Sports Med 2008;38(4):345–56.

49. Gaeta M, Minutoli F, Scribano E, et al. CT and MR imaging findings in athletes with early tibial stress injuries: comparison with bone scintigraphy findings and emphasis on cortical abnormalities. Radiology 2005;235(2):553–61.

50. Holder LE, Michael RH. The specific scintigraphic pattern of "shin splints in the lower leg": concise communication. J Nucl Med 1984;25(8):865–9.

51. AokY, Yasuda K, Tohyama H, et al. Magnetic resonance imaging in stress fractures and shin splints. Clin Orthop Relat Res 2004;(421):260–7.

52. Anderson MW, Ugalde V, Batt M, et al. Shin splints: MR appearance in a preliminary study. Radiology 1997;204(1):177–80.

53. Batt ME, Ugalde V, Anderson MW, et al. A prospective controlled study of diagnostic imaging for acute shin splints. Med Sci Sports Exerc 1998;30(11):1564–71.

54. Chisin R, Milgrom C, Giladi M, et al. Clinical significance of nonfocal scintigraphic findings in suspected tibial stress fractures. Clin Orthop Relat Res 1987;(220):200–5.

55. Nielsen MB, Hansen K, Holmer P, et al. Tibial periosteal reactions in soldiers. A scintigraphic study of 29 cases of lower leg pain. Acta Orthop Scand 1991;62(6):531–4.

56. Zwas ST, Elkanovitch R, Frank G. Interpretation and classification of bone scintigraphic findings in stress fractures. J Nucl Med 1987;28(4):452–7.

57. Matin P. Basic principles of nuclear medicine techniques for detection and evaluation of trauma and sports medicine injuries. Semin Nucl Med 1988;18(2):90–112.

58. Fredericson M, Bergman AG, Hoffman KL, et al. Tibial stress reaction in runners. Correlation of clinical symptoms and scintigraphy with a new magnetic resonance imaging grading system. Am J Sports Med 1995;23(4):472–8.

59. Arendt EA, Mubarak SJ, Griffiths HJ. The use of MR imaging in the assessment and clinical management of stress reactions of bone in high-performance athletes. Clin Sports Med 1997;16(2):291–306.

60. Bergman AG, Fredericson M, Ho C, et al. Asymptomatic tibial stress reactions: MRI detection and clinical follow-up in distance runners. AJR Am J Roentgenol 2004;183(3):635–8.

61. Gaeta M, Minutoli F, Vinci S, et al. High-resolution CT grading of tibial stress reactions in distance runners. AJR Am J Roentgenol 2006;187(3):7893–9.

62. Andrish JT, Bergfeld JA, Walheim J. A prospective study on the management of shin splints. J Bone Joint Surg Am 1974;56(8):1697–700.

63. Nissen LR, Astvad K, Madsen L. [Low-energy laser therapy in medial tibial stress syndrome]. Ugeskr Laeger 1994;156(49):7329–31.

64. Loudon JK, Dolphino MR. Use of foot orthoses and calf stretching for individuals with medial tibial stress syndrome. Foot Ankle Spec 2010;3(1):15–20.

65. Moen MH, Bongers T, Bakker EW. The additional value of a pneumatic leg brace in the treatment of recruits with medial tibial stress syndrome; a randomized study. J R Army Med Corps 2010;156(4):236–40.

66. Rompe JD, Cacchio A, Furia JP, et al. Low-energy extracorporeal shock wave therapy as a treatment for medial tibial stress syndrome. Am J Sports Med 2010;38(1):125–32.

67. Moen MH, Schipper M, Schmikli S, et al. Shockwave treatment for medial tibial stress syndrome in athletes; a prospective controlled study. Br J Sports Med 2011. [Epub ahead of print].

68. Krenner BJ. Case report: comprehensive management of medial tibial stress syndrome. J Chiropr Med 2002;1(3):122–4.

69. Wallensten R. Results of fasciotomy in patients with medial tibial syndrome or chronic anterior-compartment syndrome. J Bone Joint Surg Am 1983;65(9):1252–5.

70. Holen KJ, Engebretsen L, Grontvedt T, et al. Surgical treatment of medial tibial stress syndrome (shin splint) by fasciotomy of the superficial posterior compartment of the leg. Scand J Med Sci Sports 1995;5(1):40–3.

71. Jarvinen M, Aho H. Niittymaki S. Results of the surgical treatment of the medial tibial syndrome in athletes. Int J Sports Med 1989;10(1):55–7.

72. Detmer DE. Chronic shin splints. Classification and management of medial tibial stress syndrome. Sports Med 1986;3(6):436–46.
73. Yates B, Allen MJ. Barnes MR. Outcome of surgical treatment of medial tibial stress syndrome. J Bone Joint Surg Am 2003;85-A(10):1974–80.
74. Schwellnus MP, Jordaan G, Noakes TD. Prevention of common overuse injuries by the use of shock absorbing insoles. A prospective study. Am J Sports Med 1990; 18(6):636–41.
75. Schwellnus MP, Jordaan G. Does calcium supplementation prevent bone stress injuries? A clinical trial. Int J Sport Nutr 1992;2(2):165–74.
76. Larsen K, Weidich F, Leboeuf-Yde C. Can custom-made biomechanic shoe orthoses prevent problems in the back and lower extremities? A randomized, controlled intervention trial of 146 military conscripts. J Manipulative Physiol Ther 2002;25(5): 326–31.
77. Pope RP, Herbert RD, Kirwan JD, et al. A randomized trial of preexercise stretching for prevention of lower-limb injury. Med Sci Sports Exerc 2000;32(2):271–7.
78. Brushoj C, Larsen K, Albrecht-Beste E, et al. Prevention of overuse injuries by a concurrent exercise program in subjects exposed to an increase in training load: a randomized controlled trial of 1020 army recruits. Am J Sports Med 2008;36(4): 663–70.

Stress Fractures in Runners

Frank McCormick, MD[a], Benedict U. Nwachukwu, BA[b],
Matthew T. Provencher, MD[c],*

KEYWORDS
- Stress fracture • Military training • Long-distance running
- Runners

Stress fractures are a common cause of injury in runners.[1,2] Stress fractures represent a form of mechanical microcrack that occurs as a result of excess strain placed on weight-bearing lower extremity bones. The resultant overload leads to an accumulation of microdamage that the body is not able to heal. The resultant microfracture, if progressive, leads to an occult fracture.

Stress fractures were first described in military personnel in the 19th century.[3] Military physicians described a phenomenon, "march foot," that occurred in military recruits and essentially consisted of foot pain and swelling.[4] By the mid 20th century, however, stress fractures were increasingly reported in nonmilitary literature.[5-10] By the 1970s, stress fractures were well reported in the literature, and repetitive, high-impact activities, in particular, running and marching, were the most frequently reported causes of stress fractures.[1,11,12] There has been much interest in understanding the mechanisms and treatment for stress fractures.

Among military personnel, stress fractures are a common cause of lost training time and medical leave from duty. Similarly, in competitive runners, stress fractures are a common cause of suboptimal training and underperformance. In this article, we focus on stress fractures in runners. This article reviews the pathophysiology, risk factors, diagnosis, treatment, and prevention of stress fractures in runners.

PATHOPHYSIOLOGY

There is a spectrum of bone response to repetitive stress: normal response, stress reaction, and stress fracture. Stress reactions occur when repeated abnormal bone

There was no funding in support of this work.

The authors have nothing to disclose.

Disclaimer: The views expressed in this article are those of the authors and do not reflect the official policy or position of the Department of the Navy, Department of Defense, or the United States government.

[a] Orthopaedics Department, Massachusetts General Hospital, 55 Fruit Street, Boston, MA 02114, USA

[b] Harvard Medical School, Holmes Society, 260 Longwood Avenue, Boston, MA 02115, USA

[c] Department of Orthopaedic Surgery, Naval Medical Center San Diego, 11800 Bob Wilson Drive, San Diego, CA 92134, USA

* Corresponding author.

E-mail address: matthew.provencher@med.navy.mil

Clin Sports Med 31 (2012) 291–306

doi:10.1016/j.csm.2011.09.012

0278-5919/12/$ – see front matter Published by Elsevier Inc.

sportsmed.theclinics.com

stress without appropriate rest causes osteoclastic activity to outstrip osteoblastic activity.[13] This osteoclast/osteoblast imbalance initially results in microfractures; magnetic resonance imaging (MRI) at this stage would simply show bone marrow edema. If the imbalance (ie, repetitive stress) continues, the microfracture may progress to a true cortical break (stress fracture).

Active remodeling with frequent cell turnover occurs in cancellous bone, whereas remodeling and cell turnover in cortical bone is much slower; thus, cortical bone has a markedly higher frequency of stress fractures compared with cancellous bone. Because of these intrinsic bone qualities, physicians often categorize cortical fractures as abnormal stresses to normal bone and cancellous fractures as normal stresses on abnormal bone.

Stress fractures occurring in cancellous bone typically occur in athletes with low bone mineral density (BMD). In particular female athletes with a lower BMD, nutritional deficiencies, and hormonal irregularities have a markedly increased incidence of cancellous fractures when compared with men or other women without the aforementioned attributes. Low BMD, nutritional issues, and menstrual irregularities have been termed *the female athlete triad* when occurring together in a female athlete. This should be recognized, as it represents a potentially reversible cause for stress fractures in the female runner.

The location of the fracture within the bone is also predictive of healing and predicts the utility of surgical intervention. The distinction between compressive or tension forces within the bone fracture predicts outcome based on the Arbeitsgemeinschaft für Osteosynthesefragen Foundation principles of fracture healing. Compression stress fractures are more likely to heal with conservative measures, based on the intrinsic stability of the fracture pattern. The compressive forces allow for direct osteogenesis. In contrast, tension stress fractures are less likely to heal with conservation measures based on the lack of intrinsic stability at the fracture site. The tension forces tend to displace the fracture site, with recurrent instability and a resultant fracture gap. Thus, surgery often is indicated to provide this fracture stability, especially in high-risk fractures or for athletes desiring quicker return to activities.

RISK FACTORS

Identifying and modifying risk factors is key to the management of stress fractures. A large portion of our knowledge about risk factors for stress fractures comes from the military literature reporting on the incidence of stress fractures among recruits, cadets, trained soldiers, and Marines.[14-18] Risk factors for stress fractures are commonly categorized as intrinsic or extrinsic (**Fig. 1**).

Intrinsic

Demographic
Female sex has been most frequently associated with an increased incidence of stress fractures. In particular, female long-distance runners appear to have the highest risk for sustaining stress fractures.[19] Although long-distance running itself can predispose runners to stress fractures, it appears that the associated nutritional and menstrual irregularities seen with increased frequency in long-distance running women is the major contributor to the increased risk. Several military and nonmilitary studies of women with amenorrhea have shown greater risks for stress fractures in these women.[20-23] It is thought that in the amenorrheic female there are lower-than-normal levels of gonadotropins and subsequently low levels of estrogen. Estrogen is an osteoclast-activating factor,

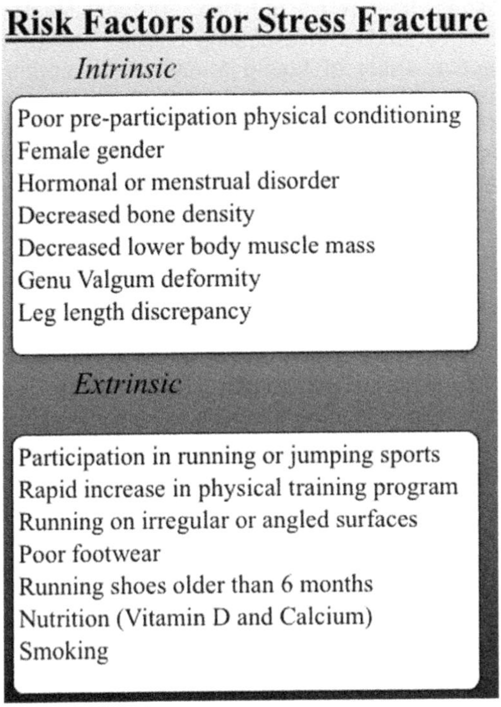

Risk Factors for Stress Fracture

Intrinsic

Poor pre-participation physical conditioning
Female gender
Hormonal or menstrual disorder
Decreased bone density
Decreased lower body muscle mass
Genu Valgum deformity
Leg length discrepancy

Extrinsic

Participation in running or jumping sports
Rapid increase in physical training program
Running on irregular or angled surfaces
Poor footwear
Running shoes older than 6 months
Nutrition (Vitamin D and Calcium)
Smoking

Fig. 1. The recognized risk factors for developing stress fractures.

and, in the amenorrheic female runner, the normal osteoclastic/osteoblastic response to repetitive stress is disrupted secondary to a lack of estrogen.

Age and race are less well-established risk factors for stress fractures. Older age and white race have been identified as potentially increasing the risk of stress fractures. The bulk of investigations on these 2 demographic risk factors have been performed on military personnel, however.[15,23–25] One nonmilitary study looked at the incidence of stress fractures among collegiate distance runners and found that white runners had a risk 2.4 times that of black runners (95% confidence interval [CI], 0.7, 8.4) and 1.9 times that of other nonwhite runners (95% CI, 1.0, 3.5).[19]

Lifestyle/behavior

Level of activity (ie, sedentary vs active) has been associated with an increased risk of stress fractures. One military study documented an increased incidence of stress fractures among recruits with lower levels of activity before military training.[24] There is a relative paucity of literature looking at similar phenomena in runners and athletes; however, one study looking at stress fractures in college athletes over a 3-year period found that 67% of stress fractures occurred in freshmen, whereas only 7% occurred among seniors.[26]

One modifiable behavior that appears to correlate well with an increased risk of stress fractures is smoking status. Several studies have found that there is a high incidence of stress fractures among smokers.[27–29]

Nutrition

Calcium and vitamin D homeostasis is becoming increasingly recognized as integral to optimal bone health. Investigators have long suggested an association between calcium intake and stress fracture risk in runners and athletes. However, there have only been 2 prospective studies investigating calcium intake and stress fracture risk.[30] One prospective study of young female cross country runners for an average of 1.85 years found significant reductions in fracture incidence and risk: fracture risk reduction of 62% for each additional cup of skim milk consumed per day.[31] The other prospective study was a randomized, controlled trial. The study was an 8-week trial of supplementation with 2000 mg calcium and 800 IU vitamin D versus no supplementation. The study found a significant 20% reduction in fracture injuries in those on supplementation.[32] On the basis of the available literature, it appears that intake of high levels of calcium (1500–2000 mg) may be protective against stress fractures.

Mechanics/anatomy

It is becoming increasingly recognized that biomechanical factors are associated with stress fracture risk. Smaller calf girth and less lower limb muscle mass has been shown to put female runners at increased risk for stress fractures.[33] It is thought that increased lower limb muscle mass helps absorb some of the forces transmitted to bone during running. This observation may partially explain why female runners, who have narrower bones than their male counterparts, are more predisposed to stress fracture. Although less well studied, it has also been suggested that kinetic and kinematic biomechanical variables can contribute to stress fracture risk. For example, it has been shown that running with excessive hip adduction and rear-foot eversion predisposes runners to tibial stress fractures.[34]

Anatomic considerations have also been found to predispose athletes to stress fractures. Studies investigating knee alignment have found valgus knees ("knock-knees") and quadriceps angle greater than 15° lead to a significantly higher cumulative incidence of stress fractures.[35,36] It has also been shown that runners with stress fractures tend to have leg length discrepancies.[19]

Extrinsic

It is well understood that the amount of training performed, regardless of other risk factors, independently increases one's risk for stress fractures. In other words, higher amounts of running are associated in general with increased risk for fractures.[37–41] However, this observation is of little therapeutic value given that one cannot predict how much running/training is sufficient for each individual athlete. It is worth noting, however, that a military study attempting to study the fitness versus amount of training paradigm found that in training units in which recruits had fewer training miles run, these recruits experienced a significantly lower incidence of stress injury but also performed as well on final fitness tests.[42] Although the absolute amount of training can pose a risk for stress fractures, it has also been suggested that insufficient rest and time for bone recovery is a bigger risk factor for the development of stress fractures. The literature is inconclusive, however, and there are studies to suggest a benefit to implementing recovery periods (ie, a "no running" period during training) as well as studies that show no benefit when recovery time is incorporated into a training regimen.

Equipment and running terrain have also been shown to affect the risk of stress fracture in runners. One study of environmental risks for stress fractures in runners found that runners with stress fractures were more likely to report a change in running surface or running on a hilly terrain.[19] A similar relationship has been documented in the military literature; a switch from marching on flat terrain to marching on hilly, rocky terrain has been shown to cause a higher incidence of stress fractures.[43]

It has also been found that a training shoe older than 6 months is a risk factor for the development of stress fracture.[24] It is thought that with time and use, training shoes lose their shock absorptive capacity, and the strain from running is more easily transmitted to bone. Shock-absorbent insoles have been found to be beneficial in protecting the feet and lower extremities from stress fracture development.[44] In particular, arch supports may prove to be of greatest benefit to runners with pes planus (flat foot).

EVALUATION

Most runners presenting with a stress fracture present to their physician with a localizable pain of insidious onset. Runners often do not recollect a specific inciting event or injury to the area. In the early presentation, the pain typically is not present at rest but occurs with runs, especially at the end of runs. If the fracture is not attended to, the runner will progress to experiencing pain at earlier parts of their run, and at a more advanced stage the runner may experience pain with rest or with routine ambulation.

It is always important to elicit history regarding predisposing factors to stress fractures. Such information can be crucial in tailoring treatment and rehabilitation protocols as well as preventing recurrence. It is important to note eating habits, menstrual history (in female runners), and training patterns (adequate rest; change in training frequency, intensity, modality, or terrain; proper use and turnover of training equipment). A recent change in training activity is a very common finding.

A thorough history is highly suggestive, and the physical examination can be confirmatory. The classic physical examination finding is reproducible focal point tenderness. Swelling and warmth can also be present at the area of tenderness. However, this is not a requisite for the diagnosis.

Imaging is often utilized to supplement the history and physical examination. The imaging of choice has become MRI. Radiographs are not primarily high yield for initial assessments, given that it can take up to 3 weeks for a stress fracture to become evident on radiograph via cortical irregularities and a periosteal reaction. Bone scans are a highly sensitive modality for diagnosing stress fractures and were traditionally used in cases of uncertainty. The major drawbacks of bone scans are that they are very time consuming and nonspecific and are a poor choice to monitor recovery, as the bone can continue to have increased uptake even after fracture healing. Bone scans have fallen out of favor since the advent of computed tomography (CT) and MRI. Both CT scans and MRIs are useful in the diagnosis of stress fractures. Compared with CT scans, MRIs provide sensitivity closer that of to bone scans and also help avoid exposing patients to radiation. Further, MRIs allow for the concurrent evaluation of soft tissue. Changes are detected by MRI weeks before changes are detected radiographically.[45,46]

An important clinical step is to determine the severity and prognosis of a stress fracture. Unfortunately, there currently is no classification system offering both validated radiographic and clinical parameters by which to grade a stress fracture.[47] Many are location specific. The Arendt and Griffiths system is the most commonly referenced system since 2000.[48] One commonly adopted general convention, which we will use in this review, is to classify stress fractures as high risk versus low risk based on the anatomic location of the fracture and the natural history of fractures occurring at this anatomic site.[49–51] This provides treatment and prognostic parameters (**Fig. 2**).

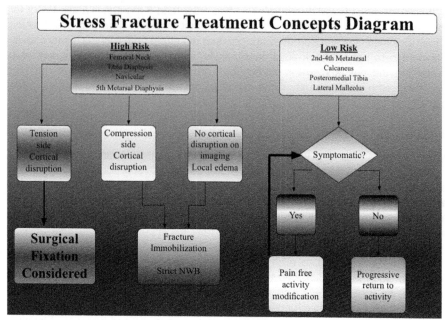

Fig. 2. General treatment concepts for stress fractures.

HIGH-RISK STRESS FRACTURES
Femoral Neck

Femoral neck stress fractures are a potential source of high morbidity in runners. The insidious nature of femoral neck stress fracture presentation combined with a low clinical suspicion commonly leads to serious complications. Reported complication rates after femoral neck stress fractures have ranged from 20% to 86%.[52–54] Possible complications include fracture completion, malunion with resultant impingement, nonunion, avascular necrosis, and arthritic changes.

Runners presenting with femoral neck stress fractures typically will describe a history of anterior hip or groin pain that worsens with activity.[55] Patients often give a history of having participated in an activity with the characteristic triad of being new, strenuous, and highly repetitive. Physical examination is often vague, with log rolling and active straight leg raises sometimes provocative. Given that plain radiographs may not always reveal a fracture until several weeks after injury, it is generally recommended to obtain an MRI if radiographs are negative, and it is reasonable to proceed directly to an MRI to screen for and rule out other possible causes of hip and groin pain.[55]

Treatment of femoral neck fractures is dictated by the location of the fracture. Fractures of the superior aspect of the femoral neck tend to be secondary to tensile forces, whereas fractures of the inferior aspect of the femoral neck tend to be secondary to compressive forces. Because tension side fractures on the superior aspect tend to be at greatest risk for displacement and subsequent complication, it is generally recommended that these fractures be managed with internal fixation.[56] The Naval Medical Center Classification[57] further characterizes compressive sided injuries on the basis of a fatigue line (**Figs. 3** and **4**). The fatigue line is an MR finding of low signal intensity lying perpendicular to femoral neck. The 3 subtypes of compression fractures are (1) no fatigue line, (2) a fatigue line of less than 50% the

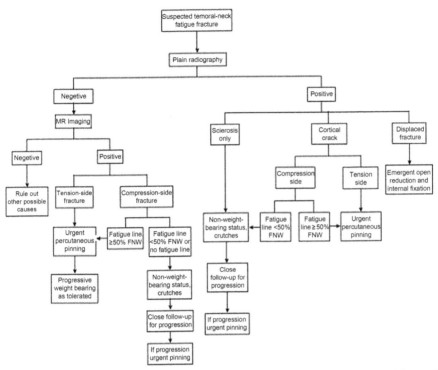

Fig. 3. Naval Medical Center San Diego classification scheme for the treatment of femoral neck stress fracture. (*From* Shin AY, Gillingham BL. Fatigue fractures of the femoral neck in athletes. J Am Acad Orthop Surg 1997;5(6):293–302; with permission. © 1997 American Academy of Orthopaedic Surgeons.)

width of the femoral neck, and (3) a fatigue line equal or greater than 50%. Treatment recommendations based on the fracture line are given in the treatment flow diagram. In conservatively treated patients, it is key to have close follow-up with repeat imaging to prevent progression and confirm resolution of fracture. Progression and then displacement of femoral neck fractures considerably increases the risk of complications.

Anterior Tibial Shaft

The tibial shaft is the most common location for stress fractures in athletes.[49] Although tibial shaft stress fractures are relatively common, most of these fractures are posteromedial and considered low risk. Only anterior tibial fractures are considered high risk. This is because of the force propagation on the tibia and healing potential. Anterior tibial stress fractures are tension-side fractures and, as such, are at risk for delayed healing and nonunion. Classically, anterior tibial shaft stress fractures present in runners as anterior leg pain or poorly localized discomfort. Physical examination of the runner with anterior tibial shaft stress fracture may reveal erythema or swelling at the site of fracture, but this is nonspecific.

Initial radiographic workup is an appropriate first step. MRI is very sensitive and allows for evaluation of the soft tissue. A "dreaded black-line" on the anterior tibia radiograph at the middle-distal third junction of the anterior tibia is pathognomonic for

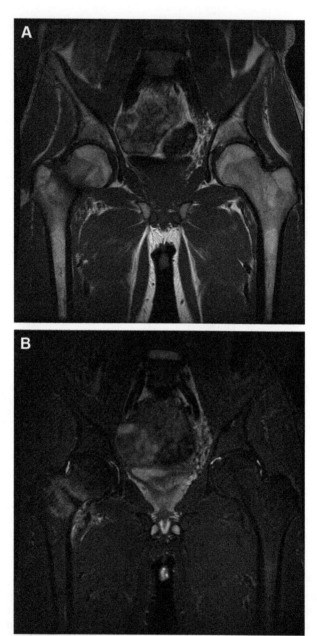

Fig. 4. (*A*) Coronal T1-weighted (repetition time [TR], 580 msec; echo time [TE], 15 msec) and (*B*) T2-weighted (TR, 2000; TE, 80) MRI show the fatigue line. T1 imaging shows a semicircular zone of decreased signal intensity centered on the posteromedial cortex of the femoral neck, representing edema extending nearly completely across the femoral neck. Within this area of low-signal intensity is a dark line of lower signal intensity extending across the femoral neck perpendicular to the cortex, consistent with a complete nondisplaced femoral-neck stress fracture. The same low-signal intensity line on the T2 imaging better shows the cortical disruption on the compression side of the bone.

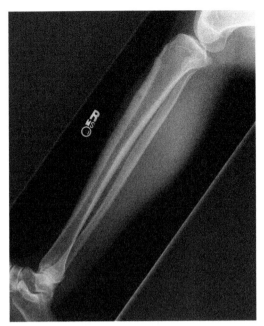

Fig. 5. Radiographs of a lateral tibia show a tibial stress fracture "dreaded black line" typically found on the anterior cortex at the middle-distal third junction with a linear lucency of cortical disruption. Identification of this radiographic parameter is a poor prognostic indicator for union and often is considered an operative indication in athletes desiring an expedited, reliable return to play.

this fracture and is an indicator for fracture completion in tension (**Fig. 5**). Many runners should be considered for surgical intervention at this point to expedite recovery and optimize outcomes. Available literature suggests that surgical management of anterior tibial shaft fractures can lead to fracture union and a return to sports of up to 5 months earlier than conservatively managed fractures.[55]

Both operative and nonoperative methods have been used effectively to treat anterior tibial shaft stress fractures.[58,59] Runners with anterior tibial stress fractures treated surgically will typically receive an intramedullary nail. This allows for immediate weight bearing and fracture site debridement and helps avoid soft tissue and periosteal dissection at the fracture site. Runners treated conservatively are treated with rest and restricted weight bearing with a gradual return to activity. This is often a more gradual return to sports.

Navicular

Navicular stress fractures are relatively frequent in runners or athletes requiring "push-off." Sprinters and middle distance runners have navicular stress fractures more commonly than long-distance runners, likely because of the high torque forces required in push off.[33] The navicular bone is highly vulnerable to stress fractures because of a relative avascularity complicated by a physical compression between the talus and the cuneiforms with load-bearing in plantar-flexion.[60] Moreover, once a fracture is incited, these components, in turn, complicate healing.

Runners with navicular fractures typically complain of vague, poorly localized foot pain, primarily over the medial dorsum of the foot. They often describe the pain as insidious and increasing with activity. A common but by no means universal finding is tenderness at the "N-spot" on the dorsal navicular. Because plain radiographs often are negative in acutely assessing for a navicular fracture, MRI has become the diagnostic tool of choice. Navicular stress fractures are often linear in the central one third.[61]

A meta-analysis investigating conservative versus surgical treatment of navicular fractures suggested that there is no advantage for surgical treatment compared with non–weight-bearing immobilization. Thus, avoiding the potential complications with surgery, the authors concluded that conservative non–weight-bearing management is the standard of care for initial treatment of stress fractures of the tarsal navicular.[62] Those that do not respond to conservative measures, including non–weight-bearing periods and immobilization, are surgical candidates. Saxena and colleagues[63] proposed categorization of navicular fracture into 3 types to guide surgical intervention: type 1 fractures are low grade and respond well to non-weight bearing immobilization for 6 weeks. Types 2 and 3 fractures represent fractures with cortical disruption into the navicular body and opposite cortex. Types 2 and 3 require surgical intervention. Surgical intervention usually consists of percutaneous fixation, with bone grafting used in the case of chronic fracture, delayed union, or nonunion.[55]

Talar Neck

Talar neck stress fractures are rare, with only a few case series described in the literature, with an incidence of 4.4 per 10,000 patient-years.[64] There usually is a classic history given by runners presenting with this fracture. The runner presenting with a talar neck fracture may complain of an inciting event such as an ankle sprain followed by ankle pain, swelling, and an inability to ambulate. In this scenario, continued pain despite adequate rehabilitation should engender a high index of suspicion for fracture of the talus. On examination, patients with talar neck fractures typically will have swelling with localized discomfort around the ankle joint.

Plain radiographs are an acceptable first step in the diagnosis and workup of talar neck fractures. However CT or MRI often will be routinely performed because of their high sensitivity and ability to evaluate the soft tissues, which, in this region, can cause common problems.

Patients with nondisplaced talar neck fractures typically have a better prognosis and can be treated conservatively with non–weight-bearing cast immobilization and reimaging until fracture resolution. Talar stress fractures that go on to completion should be managed surgically.[65] Often, surgeons may consider localized bone graft to enhance healing in this relatively avascular region. Vascular compromise leading to osteonecrosis of the talus is one of the more frequently encountered complications of talar neck fractures.

Fifth Metatarsal

Metatarsal stress fractures are thought to comprise up to 20% of stress fractures. The majority of these fractures, however, occur in the second and third metatarsal shafts, with fifth metatarsal fractures being quite rare. A runner presenting with a fifth metatarsal fracture typically will report pain with weight bearing and will also give a history of recent trauma or change in running routine or terrain.[55] Physical examination may find metatarsal tenderness to palpation or swelling. Plain radiography often is sufficient to diagnose these fractures but can be initially negative. On imaging, the location of the fracture is diagnostic and therapeutic. Fifth metatarsal stress fractures are found in the diaphysis (**Fig. 6**). This is in contrast to the Jones' fracture as well as avulsion fractures. A thin, black, cortical irregularity is often found on the lateral

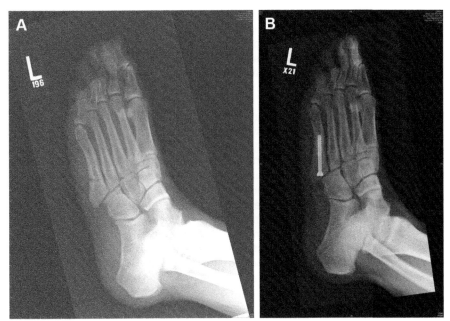

Fig. 6. (*A*) Oblique radiographs of a 19-year-old collegiate soccer player with atraumatic left foot pain during training show a linear lucency cortical disruption at the tension side of the bone. Stress fractures are commonly located at the metatarsal diaphysis. If the fracture enters the intermetatarsal joint, it is considered a Jones fracture, whereas if it enters the tarsometa-tarsal joint, it is considered an avulsion fracture. (*B*) The patient elected to undergo closed reduction and percutaneous fixation, with clinical and radiographic evidence of union at 8 weeks.

aspect of the metatarsal, at the tension side. This is a radiographic sign that signifies poor healing potential. As with other high-risk fractures, physicians should maintain a high index of suspicion and consider MRI after negative radiographs with a compelling clinical picture.

For nondisplaced fifth metatarsal fractures, 6 to 8 weeks of non–weight-bearing immobilization is generally recommended. There is a high rate of nonunion in partial weight-bearing programs. Surgery should be considered early in runners who: (1) have not responded to conservative measures or (2) have displaced fractures. Surgery is also an option for the elite runner desiring expedited return to competition.

LOW-RISK STRESS FRACTURES

Whereas high-risk stress fractures are so classified based on their tendency for incomplete healing or fracture completion, low-risk stress fractures tend to heal with conservative measures and restriction of activity only. Low-risk stress fracture sites include lateral malleolus, calcaneus, second through fourth metatarsals, and femoral shaft.

Once a low-risk stress fracture has been identified, management should be tailored to the individual runner's needs and pain symptoms. Activity modification and relative rest is typically recommended.[66] The amount of activity modification is contingent on the runner's symptoms and pain-free threshold; all activity should be titrated to a pain-free level. It is generally well supported that the reduction, not necessarily total elimination, of stress loading allows the bone to heal and repair the stress fracture while providing mechanical stimulation; hence, activity modification to a pain-free threshold is sufficient. A simple clinical guide is "if it hurts to do it, then don't do it." A runner will need to hold back intensity until the activity no longer incites pain during or afterward. In more advanced scenarios, a runner may experience pain with walking and weight bearing. In such cases, a short trial of crutch walking or non–weight bearing on the affected extremity is necessary. This will need to continue until the activity is pain free, allowing for the gentle progression of activities. To maintain fitness in competitive runners, non–weight-bearing activities, such as biking, swimming, water running, and upper-body cross training often are recommended.

With no other intervention, a runner with a low-risk stress fracture should have adequate stress fracture healing within 4 to 8 weeks of modified activity.[51] A stepwise return to activity is recommended once the runner is pain free and the fracture site is nontender. It is generally thought that athletes returning to activity after relative rest should escalate their activity by no more than 10% each week. Although there is no clear evidence supporting this recommendation, theoretically, a premature return to full activity would likely disrupt fracture healing; further, a slow return to function allows for incremental bone strengthening.

There are equivocal data on whether the utilization of modalities, such as ultrasound scan and electrical stimulation during the rehabilitation period decreases healing time.[55] Ice compresses and analgesics can provide symptomatic pain relief.

TREATMENT AND PREVENTION STRATEGY

The best form of treatment for stress fractures is prevention. The astute health care provider can often identify risk factors and training errors predisposing to stress fractures. We briefly outline common risks for stress injuries and prevention modalities.

Poor bone mineral density is a very common cause of stress fractures. As mentioned earlier, a cancellous bone stress fracture should immediately alert the health care provider to investigate bone mineral density. Often, because distance runners aim to maintain lean body mass, they are at increased risk for inadequate nutritional intake. It is always important to screen runners, especially if their clinical appearance is suggestive for nutritional imbalance. In particular, high levels of calcium (1500–2000 mg) and vitamin D supplementation appear to be protective against the development of stress fractures. Other interventions that should be considered in addressing poor bone mineral density include smoking cessation and weight loss.

Poor training regimens and old training equipment are easily modifiable risk factors for stress fractures, which an astute health care provider can screen for and either prevent a stress injury or prevent recurrence. The role of footwear modification in stress fracture genesis has been well studied in the military literature. A reasonable conclusion based on the literature is that frequent footwear change (every 6 months or 300–500 miles) is essential and also that certain shock-absorbent materials (eg, in-soles) can independently decrease the risk of stress fractures.[44]

Over the last decade, bisphosphonates have gained in popularity for the treatment of a number of bone diseases. The potential role of bisphosphonates has been considered in the treatment and prevention of stress fractures. As explained earlier, stress loading of bone initiates a remodeling and continued loading that progresses to an early stress fracture if the bone is not allowed time to heal. Animal models have suggested that use of bisphosphonates may delay fracture maturation and further progression to an advanced stress fracture. However, given the side-effect profile for bisphosphonates, well-constructed, controlled trials are needed to better characterize the risk–benefit of using bisphosphonates in the prevention and treatment of stress fractures.[67]

SUMMARY

Stress fractures are a relatively common entity in athletes, in particular, runners. Physicians and health care providers should maintain a high index of suspicion for stress fractures in runners presenting with insidious onset of focal bone tenderness associated with recent changes in training intensity or regimen. It is particularly important to recognize "high-risk" fractures, as these are associated with an increased risk of complication. A patient with confirmed radiographic evidence of a high-risk stress fracture should be evaluated by an orthopedic surgeon. Runners may benefit from orthotics, cushioned sneakers, interval training, and vitamin/calcium supplementation as a means of stress fracture prevention.

REFERENCES

1. Matheson GO, Clement DB, Mckenzie DC, et al. Stress fractures in athletes. A study of 320 cases. Am J Sports Med 1987;15(1):46–58.
2. McBryde AM Jr. Stress fractures in athletes. J Sports Med 1975;3:212–7.
3. Breithaupt J. Zur pathologie des menschlichen fussess. Medizin Zeitung 1855;24: 169–77.
4. Jansen M. March foot. J Bone Joint Surg Am 1926;8:262–72.
5. Burrows H, Fatigue fracture of the middle third of the tibia in ballet dancers. J Bone Joint Surg 1956;38B:83–94.
6. Devas MB. Stress fractures of the tibia in athletes or "Shin soreness." J Bone Joint Surg 1958;40B:227–39.
7. Hartley JB. Fatigue fracture of the tibia. Br J Surg 1943;30:9–14.
8. Blazina ME, Watanabe RS, Drake EC. Fatigue fracture in track athletes. Calif Med 1962;97:61–3.
9. Berkebile RD. Stress fracture of the tibia in children. Am J Roentgenol 1964;91: 588–96.
10. Devas MB. Stress fractures in athletes. Proc R Soc Med 1969;62:933–7.
11. Belkin SC. Stress fractures in athletes. Orthop Clin North Am 1980;11:735–62.
12. Hukko A, Alen M, Orava S. Stress fractures of the lower leg. Scand J Sports Med Sci 1987;9:1–8.
13. Beck BR. Tibial stress injuries. An aetiological review for the purposes of guiding management. Sports Med 1998;26(4):265–79.
14. Linenger JM, Shwayhat AF. Epidemiology of podiatric injuries in U.S. Marine recruits undergoing basic training. J Am Podiatr Med Assoc 1992;82:269–71.
15. Brudvig TJ, Gudger TD, Obermeyer L. Stress fractures in 295 trainees: a one year study of incidence as related to age, sex, and race. Mil Med 1983;148: 666–7.
16. Jones BH, Bovee MW, Harris JM 3rd, et al. Intrinsic risk factors for exercise-related injuries among male and female army trainees. Am J Sports Med 1993;2(5):705–10.
17. Beck TJ, Shaffer RA, Betsinger K, et al. Stress fracture in military recruits: gender differences in muscle and bone susceptibility factors. Bone 2000;27(3):437–44.
18. Protzman RR, Griffis CC. Comparative stress fracture incidence in males and females in an equal training environment. Athletic Train 1971;121:126–31.
19. Brunet ME, Cook SD, Brinker MR, et al. A survey of running injuries in 1505 competitive and recreational runners. J Sports Med Phys Fitness 1990;30(3):307–15.
20. Lloyd T, Triantafyllou SJ, Baker ER, et al. Women athletes with menstrual irregularity have increased musculoskeletal injuries. Med Sci Sports Exerc 1986;18(4):374–9.

21. Barrow GW, Saha S. Menstrual irregularity and stress fractures in collegiate female distance runners. Am J Sports Med 1988;16:209–16.
22. Myburgh KH, Hutchins J, Fataar AB, et al. Low bone density is an etiologic factor for stress fractures in athletes. Ann Intern Med 1990;113(10):754–9.
23. Friedl KE, Nuovo JA, Patience TH, et al. Factors associated with stress fracture in young army women: indications for further research. Mil Med 1992;157(7):334–8.
24. Gardner LI Jr, Dziados JE, Jones BH, et al. Prevention of lower extremity stress fractures: a controlled trial of a shock absorbent insole. Am J Public Health 1988; 78(12):1563–7.
25. Shaffer RA, Brodine SK, Almeida SA, et al. Use of simple measures of physical activity to predict stress fractures in young men undergoing a rigorous physical training program. Am J Epidemiol 1999;149(3):236–42.
26. Goldberg B, Pecora P. Stress fractures: a risk of increased training in freshmen. Phys Sports Med 1994;22:68–78.
27. Altarac M, Gardner JW, Popovich RM, et al. Cigarette smoking and exercise-related injuries among young men and women. Am J Prev Med 2000;18:96–102.
28. Jones BH, Cowan DN, Tomlinson JP, et al. Epidemiology of injuries associated with physical training among young men in the army. Med Sci Sports Exerc 1993;25(2): 197–203.
29. Reynolds KL, Keckel HA, Witt CE, et al. Cigarette smoking, physical fitness, and injuries in infantry soldiers. Am J Prev Med 1994;10(3):145–50.
30. Tenforde AS, Sayres LC, Sainani KL, et al. Evaluating the relationship of calcium and vitamin d in the prevention of stress fracture injuries in the young athlete: a review of the literature. Phys Med Rehabil 2010;2:945–9.
31. Nieves JW, Melsop K, Curtis M, et al. Nutritional factors that influence change in bone density and stress fracture risk among young female cross-country runners. Phys Med Rehabil 2010;2:740–50.
32. Lappe J, Cullen D, Haynatzki G, et al. Calcium and vitamin D supplementation decreases incidence of stress fractures in female navy recruits. J Bone Miner Res 2008;23:741–9.
33. Bennell KL, Malcolm SA, Thomas SA, et al. The incidence and distribution of stress fractures in competitive track and field athletes. A twelve-month prospective study. Am J Sports Med 1996;24(2):211–7.
34. Pohl MB, Mullineaux DR, Milner CE, et al. Biomechanical predictors of retrospective tibial stress fractures in runners. J Biomech 2008;41(6):1160–5.
35. Cowan DN, Jones BH, Frykman PN, et al. Lower limb morphology and risk of overuse injury among male infantry trainees. Med Sci Sports Exerc 1996;28(8):945–52.
36. Finestone A, Shlamkovitch N, Eldad A, et al. Risk factors for stress fractures among Israeli infantry recruits. Mil Med 1991;156(10):528–30.
37. Jones BH, Cowan DN, Knapik JJ. Exercise, training and injuries. Sports Med 1994;18:202–14.
38. Gilchrist J, Jones BH, Sleet DA, et al. Exercise-related injuries among women: strategies for prevention from civilian and military studies. MMWR Recomm Rep 2000;49(RR–2):15–33.
39. Koplan JP, Powell KE, Sikes RK, et al. An epidemiologic study of the benefits and risks of running. JAMA 1982;248(23):3118–21.
40. Macera CA, Pate RR, Powell KE, et al. Predicting lower-extremity injuries among habitual runners. Arch Intern Med 1989;149(11):2565–8.
41. Marti B, Vader JP, Minder CE, et al. On the epidemiology of running injuries. The 1984 Bern Grand-Prix study. Am J Sports Med 1988;16(3):285–94.

42. Jones BH, Shaffer RA, Snedecor MR. Injuries treated in out-patient clinics: surveys and research data. Mil Med 1999;164(Suppl):6–89.
43. Zahger D, Abrmovitz A, Zellikovsky L, et al. Stress fractures in female soldiers: an epidemiological investigation of an outbreak. Mil Med 1988;153(9):448–50.
44. Jones BH, Thacker SB, Gilchrist J, et al. Prevention of lower extremity stress fractures in athletes and soldiers: a systematic review. Epidemiol Rev 2002;24(2):228–47.
45. Lee JK, Yao L. Stress fractures: MR imaging. Radiology 1988;169(1):217–20.
46. Spitz DJ, Newberg AH. Imaging of stress fractures in the athlete. Clin North Am 2002;40(2):313–31.
47. Miller T, Kaeding CC, Flanigan D. The classification systems of stress fractures: a systematic review. Phys Sports Med 2011;39(1):93–100.
48. Arendt EA, Griffiths HJ. The use of mr imaging in the assessment and clinical management of stress reactions of bone in high-performance athletes. Clin Sports Med 1997;16(2):291–306.
49. Boden BP, Osbahr DC. High-risk stress fracture: evaluation and treatment. J Am Acad Orthop Surg 2000;6:344–53.
50. Boden BP, Osbahr DC, Jimenez C. Low-risk stress fractures. Am J Sports Med 2001;29(1):100–11.
51. Brukner P, Bradshaw C, Bennell K. Managing common stress fractures: let risk level guide treatment. Sports Med 1998;26(8):39–47.
52. Lee CH, Huang GS, Chao KH, et al. Surgical treatment of displaced stress fractures of the femoral neck in military recruits: a report of 42 cases. Arch Orthop Trauma Surg 2003;123(1):527–33.
53. Johansson C, Ekenman I, Tornkvist H, et al. Stress fractures of the femoral neck in athletes. The consequence of a delay in diagnosis. Am J Sports Med 1990;18(5):524–8.
54. Visuri T. Stress osteopathy of the femoral head. 10 military recruits followed for 5–11 years. Acta Orthop Scand 1997;68(2):138–41.
55. Harrast MA, Colonno D. Stress fractures in runners. Clin Sports Med 2010;29(3):399–416.
56. Egol KA, Koval KJ, Kummer F, et al. Stress fractures of the femoral neck. Clin Orthop Relat Res 1998;348:72–8.
57. Shin AY, Gillingham BL. Fatigue fractures of the femoral neck in athletes. J Am Acad Orthop Surg 1997;5(6):293–302.
58. Rettig AC, Shelbourne KD, McCarroll JR, et al. The natural history and treatment of delayed union stress fractures of the anterior cortex of the tibia. Am J Sports Med 1988;16(3):250–5.
59. Stewart GW, Brunet ME, Manning MR, et al. Treatment of stress fractures in athletes with intravenous pamidronat. Clin J Sport Med 2005;15(2):92–4.
60. Golano P, Farinas O, Saenz I. The anatomy of the navicular and periarticular structures. Foot Ankle Clin 2004;9(1):1–23.
61. Korpelainen R, Orava S, Karpakka J, et al. Risk factors for recurrent stress fractures in athletes. Am J Sports Med 2001;29(3):304–10.
62. Torg JS, Moyer J, Gaughan JP, et al. Management of tarsal navicular stress fractures: conservative versus surgical treatment: a meta-analysis. Am J Sports Med 2010;38(5):1048–53.
63. Saxena A, Fullem B, Hannaford D. Results of treatment of 22 navicular stress fractures and a new proposed radiographic classification system. J Foot Ankle Surg 2000;39(2):96–103.
64. Sormaala MJ, Niva MH, Kiuru MJ, et al. Bone stress injuries of the talus in military recruits. Bone 2006;39(1):199–204.

65. Pajenda G, Vecsei V, Reddy B, et al. Treatment of talar neck fractures: clinical results of 50 patients. J Foot Ankle Surg 2000;39(6):365–75.
66. Kaeding CC, Najarian RG. Stress fractures: classification and management. Phys Sports Med 2010;38(3):45–54.
67. Shima Y, Engebretsen L, Junji I, et al. Use of bisphosphonates for the treatment of stress fractures in athletes. Knee Surg Sports Traumatol Arthrosc 2009;17(5):542–50.

Chronic Exertional Compartment Syndrome

Christopher A. George, MD, Mark R. Hutchinson, MD*

KEYWORDS

- Chronic exertional compartment syndrome
- Leg pain in athletes • Compartment pressure • Fasciotomy

Exercise-related leg pain is a frequent problem seen in recreational and competitive athletes. There is a broad differential in the diagnosis of leg pain in athletes; however, the majority is related to overuse. Chronic exertional compartment syndrome (CECS) is a relatively common cause of leg pain with an incidence ranging from 27% to 33%, second only to medial tibial stress syndrome (13%–42%).[1,2] Chronic exertional compartment syndrome is defined as reversible ischemia within a closed fibro-osseous space, which leads to decreased tissue perfusion and ischemic pain. CECS is often recurrent and associated with repetitive physical activity. It is most commonly seen in athletes, with a particularly high incidence in runners as well as athletes in jumping and cutting sports. Despite the predominance of CECS in athletes, it can also occur in nonathletes or sedentary individuals who have activity-related leg pain.[3] The diagnosis should also be considered in diabetic patients with activity-related leg pain, especially in the absence of claudication symptoms.[4] Pain symptoms occur at an exertion level at which the elevation in pressure exceeds the rate of metabolism. The tissues, in turn, become tight and painful. The pain typically disappears quickly with rest, and no permanent damage to the tissue within the compartment occurs. In rare cases when an athlete continues to compete through pain, CECS can convert to an irreversible acute compartment syndrome.

The first report of CECS was by Mavor in 1956,[5] where a soccer player was successfully treated with fasciotomy and was able to return to sport. Other reports published in the 1960s and 1970s continued to highlight the clinical features of CECS and, importantly, the good results seen with early surgical intervention.[6,7] There has been continued progress in the diagnosis and treatment of CECS over the last decades.

CECS is a distinct condition from acute compartment syndrome. Acute compartment syndrome is associated with a traumatic event, and patients present with severe

The authors have nothing to disclose.
Department of Orthopaedic Surgery, University of Illinois Hospital at Chicago, 835 South Wolcott Avenue, M/C 844, Chicago, IL 60612, USA
* Corresponding author.
E-mail address: mhutch@uic.edu

Box 1
Structures within each anatomic compartment of the lower leg

Anterior

   Tibialis anterior muscle

   Extensor hallucis longus muscle

   Extensor digitorum longus muscle

   Peroneus tertius muscle

   Deep peroneal nerve

   Anterior tibial artery and vein

Lateral

   Peroneus longus muscle

   Peroneus brevis muscle

   Superficial peroneal nerve

Superficial posterior

   Gastrocnemius muscle

   Soleus muscle

   Sural nerve

Deep posterior

   Flexor hallucis longus muscle

   Flexor digitorum longus muscle

   Tibialis posterior muscle

   Posterior tibial nerve

   Posterior tibial artery and vein

pain that is worsened with passive stretch of the muscles that does not improve with rest. Acute compartment syndrome requires emergent surgical intervention to prevent limb ischemia and permanent tissue damage.

The area most commonly affected by CECS is the lower leg. It can also occur in other locations and has been described in the thigh and forearm. This review will concentrate on the lower leg, as it is the most common area; however, the clinical features, diagnosis, and treatment strategies are similar for all locations.

ANATOMY

The lower leg is divided into 4 compartments: anterior, lateral, superficial posterior, and deep posterior (**Box 1**). In addition to the respective muscles in each compartment, they all contain 1 major nerve, and 2 of the compartments contain a major blood vessel. The anterior compartment contains the deep peroneal nerve and the anterior tibial artery. The lateral compartment contains the superficial peroneal nerve. The superficial posterior compartment contains the sural nerve. The deep posterior compartment contains the posterior tibial nerve and the posterior tibial artery.

The anterior compartment is most commonly affected in CECS (45%), followed by the deep posterior compartment (40%).[8] Less commonly affected are the lateral

(10%) and superficial posterior compartments (5%).[8] In addition to a tight compartment and pain, the associated symptoms the patient reports are related directly to the contents of the affected compartment.

PATHOPHYSIOLOGY

With physical activity, normal muscle physiology and response can lead to a 20% increase in muscle volume.[9] Volume expansion within noncompliant fascial and osseous boundaries leads to an increase in the pressure within the compartment. After a certain pressure threshold, the blood flow becomes insufficient for the metabolic requirements of the muscle, and individuals begin experiencing pain. The most physiologic and representative intracompartmental pressures are obtained when the muscle is in a noncontractile state, as muscles receive blood flow during the relaxation phase, which may, in turn, artificially elevate the pressures. Patients will continue to experience pain until the intracompartmental pressure decreases to the level in which blood flow can again meet physiologic demands. This typically requires cessation of activity and a period of rest.

Anatomic variations can also play a significant role in the incidence of CECS. Fascial defects of the anterolateral leg have been observed in up to 40% of individuals with CECS, compared with less than 5% of asymptomatic individuals.[10] These fascial rents may represent the body's attempt to accomplish an auto release, or the muscle herniation may be a source of pain in and of themselves. The most common location of fascial defect is near the intramuscular septum of the anterior and lateral compartments, at the exit of the superficial peroneal nerve. The nerve may be compressed by the edge of the defect or secondary to bulging of the muscle. During exercise, a palpable bulge may be felt, and localized tenderness may occur.

Other factors may contribute to the symptoms and pathology of CECS, beyond the concept of restricted compartment expansion. Muscle herniation cannot be the pain source for all patients, as fascial rents are not always visualized in pressure-positive CECS. Of special interest, total intramuscular pressure often remains more elevated than in normal individuals even after fasciotomy, suggesting some other source of pathophysiology.[11] A study by Edmundsson and colleagues[12] found that patients with CECS have a lower capillary density and a lower number of capillaries in relation to muscle fiber size compared with controls. This lower capillary supply decreases the structural capacity of muscle blood flow, and they propose the low capillarity as a key part of the pathogenesis of CECS. Arteriolar regulation and blood flow may also play a role.

EVALUATION

A thorough and detailed history is paramount in the evaluation of patients with suspected CECS. Patients classically have no pain or symptoms while at rest. Typical patients with CECS are athletes, commonly runners, who are less than 30 years old. The characteristic complaint is recurrent, exercise-induced pain that occurs at a well-defined and reproducible point during exercise.[13]

Pain often begins as a dull aching or burning over the involved compartment and increases to the point at which exercise must be stopped. A majority of patients present with bilateral symptoms, There is an equal incidence between males and females.[14] Affected individuals are able to reliably predict the duration or intensity of exercise where symptoms will occur as well as how long the pain will last after cessation of exercise. The period of rest before resolution tends to increase in length as the symptoms become more severe. There is generally no history of trauma or

Table 1		
Differential diagnosis of leg pain in athletes		
Diagnosis	Distinctive Features	Diagnostic Studies
Stress fracture	Localized pain directly over tibia Recent increase in activity level	Bone scan, MRI
Medial tibial stress syndrome	Pain along posteromedial border of tibia Diffuse pain along length of tibia	Bone scan, MRI
Peripheral nerve entrapment	Tingling and numbness in a specific anatomic distribution	EMG, NCV
Popliteal artery entrapment	Pain and cool sensation in limb Paradoxical claudication	Angiogram

injury at the onset of symptoms. Symptoms tend to recur even after a period of discontinuation from their sport.

Physical examination of the extremity at rest is typically normal. Re-examination after an exercise challenge is necessary for a complete examination. After exercise, the affected compartment may reveal tenderness and increased tension. Palpation of the leg may identify an area of muscle herniation, typically at the junction of the middle and distal one-third of the leg. A thorough neurologic examination will identify paresthesias or areas of decreased sensation related to the nerve traversing the involved compartment. Muscle weakness can be appreciated in severe cases, and atrophy may be present in unilateral cases.

Many other conditions cause leg pain in athletes and should be considered in the differential diagnosis during evaluation (Table 1). A thorough history and physical examination should consider stress fractures, especially when the history, physical examination, and diagnostic measurement findings are not consistent with CECS, and further testing should be considered to evaluate for these other conditions. Indeed, overlapping diagnoses can occasionally occur. Stress fracture leading to periosteal and soft tissue swelling may become just enough of a trigger to throw a previously asymptomatic patient into a symptomatic CECS. The underlying pathology must be identified and addressed to assure a successful outcome.

DIAGNOSTIC TESTING

Similar to acute compartment syndrome, the diagnosis of CECS is largely clinical. When objective data are desired, measurement of intracompartmental pressure should be completed. Measurement of pressure during exercise is difficult. Postexercise and resting measurements are the standard for confirmation of the diagnosis. Some investigators also recommend a delayed measurement of intra-articular pressures 10 minutes after exercises. The type and duration of exercise before measurement must be sufficient to provoke the onset of pain symptoms. The senior author routinely recommends that the athlete continue his stress exercise 5 minutes into their pain to assure a diagnostic measurement. There has been some clinical debate regarding whether the examiner should routinely test all 4 compartments or only the symptomatic compartment. The advantage of testing an isolated compartment is that the testing is quicker and does not subject the patient to undue trauma of additional needle sticks. The advantage of routinely testing all 4 compartments is the assurance that any elevations in adjacent compartments can be identified and treated, thus reducing the risk of recurrence or surgical failure. The senior author always tests all 4

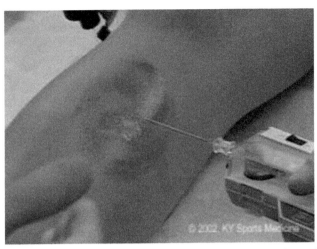

Fig. 1. The mid-medial aspect of the right leg is prepared with Betadine. The hand-held compartment pressure-testing device (Stryker Corporation, Kalamazoo, MI, USA) is in position to assess the pressures in the deep posterior compartment. (*Courtesy of* Mary Lloyd Ireland and Kentucky Sports Medicine.)

compartments both before and after exertion in an effort to optimize outcomes and avoid recurrence.

Many different methods have been described for measuring compartment pressure, including needle manometer,[15] slit catheter,[16] microtip pressure method,[17] wick catheter,[18] and microcapillary infusion.[19] Assuming correct techniques for each, they show equal effectiveness in pressure measurement. The Stryker Intracompartmental Pressure Monitor (Stryker Corp, Kalamazoo, MI, USA) is a convenient, hand-held, battery-operated device that is easy to use in the clinical setting (**Fig. 1**). Use of this particular monitor has shown good reproducibility between examiners.[20] Other commercially available monitors may be equally effective but have not been used routinely by the senior author.

The pressure criteria described by Pedowitz and colleagues[21] have been generally accepted in the diagnosis of CECS. One of the following criteria must be met in addition to a consistent history and physical examination. A resting, pre-exercise pressure greater than or equal to 15 mm Hg; 1-minute postexercise pressure greater than or equal to 30 mm Hg; 5-minute postexercise pressure greater than or equal to 20 mm Hg. The pressure may remain elevated for 30 minutes or longer in patients with CECS. The senior author routinely measures intracompartmental pressures both before and immediately after exertion. In addition to the absolute measures noted above, an elevation in a single compartment of greater than 10 mm Hg is also considered diagnostic. We have not routinely performed a delayed measure as the pre- and immediate postmeasurements are usually diagnostic, and we do not have to subject the patient to the additional trauma of additional needle sticks. Additionally, the criteria of Whitesides and Heckman[22] in acute compartment syndrome has been applied to CECS. Critical compartment ischemia occurs when the compartment pressure increases to within 20 mm Hg of the diastolic pressure.

Care must be taken during pressure measurement. Several factors may affect the accuracy of measurement. These include use of proper equipment, position of the extremity during measurement, correct and consistent location when measuring pressure, consistent orientation of the measuring device, and proper depth of needle insertion. The limb should be placed in a relaxed and consistent position for accurate and reproducible measurements. Measurement of pressure in the anterior, lateral, and superficial posterior compartments is relatively simple. However, the deep posterior compartment is more challenging, as the exact location of the needle tip may vary. There is no universally accepted protocol for pressure measurement, and debate still exists regarding the optimal way to carry out pressure measurements.[23,24] Perhaps the most important factor is that pre- and postexertional measurements are obtained in exactly the same way, at the same location, and with the needle oriented in the same direction.

Some investigators have advocated the use of ultrasound scan during pressure measurements as a guide to consistent needle placement.[25] Peck and colleagues[26] showed no statistical difference in the use of palpation or ultrasound guidance for needle placement when testing the superficial posterior or deep posterior compartments. They recommend that use of ultrasound guidance for compartment testing be reserved for specific circumstances, such as in patients taking anticoagulant medications, patients with a large body habitus, or patients with distorted anatomy, such as that seen after trauma or surgery.

There has been increased interest in the use of alternative methods in testing for elevated compartment pressure. Near-infrared spectroscopy and MRI have shown promising results. Near-infrared spectroscopy shows deoxygenation of muscle during exercise and delayed reoxygenation postexercise in patients with CECS.[27,28] With the use of MRI, the affected compartment shows increased signal intensity on T2-weighted sequence during exercise. Failure of the compartment to return to baseline appearance within 25 minutes after exercise is considered diagnostic of CECS.[29,30] Other modalities can be used to evaluate for other conditions in the differential of CECS, including triple-phase bone scans and single-photon emission computed tomography scans.[30,31] These are best used to diagnose reactive or active bony processes, such as medial tibial stress syndrome or stress fractures.

TREATMENT

Initial management of CECS should start with conservative methods. A treatment plan generally includes reduction or cessation of inciting activities, anti-inflammatory medication, stretching, foot orthotics (when appropriate), and introduction of an alternative exercise program. Conservative measures are continued for a period of 6 to 12 weeks before recommending more aggressive treatment. Nonsurgical management typically is successful only with stoppage or significant reduction in athletic activity. However, the majority of patients with CECS who seek treatment are not willing to give up athletic activity, and an expedited timeline to surgical intervention is often considered.

Subcutaneous fasciotomy of the involved compartment remains the foundation of surgical treatment.[32] Fasciotomy can be successful in relieving pain and allowing for return to full activity in 90% of patients.[33] Multiple surgical techniques have been described in the treatment of CECS. Regardless of technique, when a fascial herniation is present, it must be included in the release for successful outcomes.

Single and double incision techniques have been described. The single incision technique uses a centrally based incision to release the fascia both proximally and distally. Dual incision techniques use 2 smaller incisions at the proximal and distal end of the limb, with the intervening fascia incised using Metzenbaum scissors or a fasciotome. For anterolateral compartment release, the superficial peroneal nerve should be visualized in the distal incision and protected during release. On the posteromedial side, the compartments should be released directly off the posterior

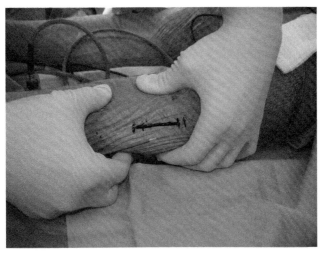

Fig. 2. The examiner can best identify the raphe between the anterior and lateral compartments of the leg by placing his fingers on the medial edge of the lateral compartment (just lateral to the anterior border of the tibia) and the posterior edge of the lateral compartment (superficial to the fibula). A gentle squeeze will display an indentation (*marked with blue marker*), which is the raphe between the anterior and lateral compartments. (*Courtesy of* Mark R. Hutchinson, MD.)

border of the tibia to avoid neurovascular injury. The structure at greatest risk of injury in the lateral approach is the superficial branch of the peroneal nerve. The structure at greatest risk of injury on the medial side is the saphenous vein or its branches. Minimal incision techniques have also been described, which use multiple small incisions to accomplish compartment release.[34] Some surgeons have advocated a combination of techniques, with a dual incision for anterolateral release and single incision for posteromedial release.

Endoscopically assisted fasciotomy is an alternative technique, which has been shown to be as safe and effective as open fasciotomy.[35,36] Advantages of endoscopic techniques are access to the entire length of the compartment and visualization of the superficial peroneal nerve and other anatomic structures that are at risk during surgical release.[35,37]

Authors Preferred Technique

The senior author (MH) uses a minimal incision, endoscopically assisted technique for fascial release. On the lateral leg, the raphe between the anterior and lateral compartments is identified (**Fig. 2**) and 2, vertical 2- to 3-cm skin incisions are made along the line of the raphe. The raphe can be identified in most patients by placing the examiners fingers on the anterior edge of the anterior compartment with the thumb on the posterior edge of the lateral compartment. A gentle squeeze creates vertical, linear indentation in the skin, which represents the adherent underlying raphe. The first lateral incision is located approximately 5 cm above the lateral malleolus directly over where the superficial peroneal exits from deep in the fascia to superficial. The second lateral incision is placed approximately 10 to 15 cm proximal to the distal wound and in line with the raphe. The medial incision is placed 1 to 2 cm posteromedial to the palpable posteromedial border of the tibia. On the medial side, subcutaneous tissue is dissected carefully down to the level of the fascia; the saphenous vein is identified and protected followed by release of the fascial attachments off the posterior medial border of the tibia. Care must be taken to control all bleeders during the procedure to reduce the risk of postoperative hematoma. A tourniquet is not necessary; indeed, we choose not to use one so that we can identify any and all bleeders at the time of surgery.

For the lateral aspect of the leg, a subcutaneous tunnel is created just above the level of the fascia both anterior and posterior to the raphe. Care must be taken not to go directly through the raphe because most penetrating vessels are located at the raphe, and aggressive dissection or retraction can lead to bleeding. Through the distal lateral incision, the superficial peroneal nerve is carefully identified and protected. It should be noted that there is a wide anatomic variation of the nerve, with some being isolated exiting the lateral compartment, some rarely exiting the anterior compartment, and many having multiple branches. If all branches are not protected, the patient may complain of postoperative paresthesias on the dorsal aspect of their foot. Once the nerve is protected, the anterior and lateral compartments are incised on either side of the intermuscular septum. Long blunt scissors or a fasciotome are used to push cut the fascia both proximally and distally. The proximal and distal 4 to 5 cm of fascia can usually be performed under direct visualization. A straight 30° angle rigid endoscope is inserted into the proximal incision above the level of the fascia. With the skin and subcutaneous tissue retracted, endoscopic visualization is used to advance the fasciotomy from distal to proximal (**Fig. 3**). The deep and superficial posterior compartments are always released under direct visualization secondary to the high risk of postoperative hematoma. Care is taken to avoid injury to the saphenous vein, which is commonly encountered lying in the groove at the insertion of the fascia onto the medial border of the tibia. The underlying muscle is again bluntly dissected from the undersurface of the fascia, and the blunt scissors are advanced proximally and

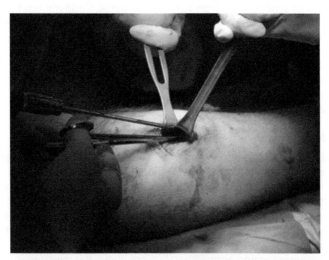

Fig. 3. Intraoperative image shows a fascial release being performed with endoscopic assistance. The wound is being held open with a single retractor, the arthroscopic serves as both a source of visualization and illumination, and the extra-long Metzenbaum scissors are used to perform the release under direct or arthroscopic visualization. (*Courtesy of* Mark R. Hutchinson, MD.)

distally to perform the fasciotomy, with the endoscope used to assist with visualization of the proximal and distal portions of the fasciotomy. While using endoscopic assistance, when a nerve, vessel, or other transverse structure is identified, the scissors should be redirected to pass either parallel to or underneath the structure. In porcine studies in our laboratory, we determined that 80% release of the length of the fascia accounts for 100% decompression of the intra-articular pressure elevation.

Clinical debate exists regarding the need to release all 4 compartments in every case or to target the affected compartment alone. Schepsis and colleagues[38] showed that in cases of isolated anterior compartment involvement, release of only the anterior compartment had equivalent results to release of the anterior and lateral compartments. Preoperative testing, including compartment pressure measurement, is critical in identifying the affected compartment(s) and planning for appropriate surgical release. In the early phases of our clinical experience, we chose to release all 4 compartments in all patients in an effort to reduce the risk of postoperative recurrence. We found an increased risk of postoperative hematoma or cellulitis in this group when compared with unilateral releases. Subsequently, we have routinely performed unilateral releases indicated by preoperative intracompartmental measurements. If the anterior or lateral compartment were elevated, then both were released. If only the deep compartment was elevated, then only a posterior medial approach was performed. This protocol significantly reduced our risk of complications.

The immediate postoperative period is aimed at pain control and limiting swelling. Compressive wraps, ice, and elevation are used in the first few days after surgery. Full weight bearing is allowed immediately after surgery; however, crutches are typically used for a short period. Active and passive range of motion exercises should also be initiated immediately after surgery to limit scarring of the released fascia. Patients should be asked to actively plantarflex their ankles and use a towel to assist full dorsiflexion. Full return to activity is generally accomplished within 8 to 12 weeks. This may be delayed if complications of postoperative hematoma or cellulites occur. For this reason, 3 days of perioperative antibiotics are recommended as well as the use of cryotherapy to reduce swelling, pain, and the risk of postoperative hematoma.

There is a lack of postoperative rehabilitation guidelines for CECS in the literature. A specific rehabilitation protocol has been proposed by Schubert,[39] which takes into consideration the duration of tissue healing, muscle loading, scar tissue formation, and consideration of all tissues contained in the involved compartment. Continued work on understanding the specifics of postoperative rehabilitation may reduce the risk of reoccurrence and optimize outcomes after fasciotomy.

OUTCOMES

There are no controlled trials in the literature that directly compare surgical and nonsurgical treatment. Similarly, there are no studies comparing the different surgical techniques.

Surgical treatment for CECS is associated with high levels of pain relief and patient satisfaction. Successful outcomes have been reported in 80% to 100% of patients.[14,32,33,38,40] However, when compartments are evaluated individually, success rates are markedly better for the anterior compartment compared with the deep posterior compartment. Successful release of the deep posterior compartment ranges from 50% to 65%.[32,38,40] This difference has been attributed to incomplete or neglected release of the deep posterior compartment. Involvement of the deep posterior compartment may also be multifactorial, and fasciotomy may not fully relieve all symptoms.[38] Endoscopic techniques have also shown excellent results, with patient satisfaction and return to preoperative activity in greater than 90% of patients.[35,36] The senior author has a series of endoscopic-assisted fasciotomies that were evaluated at 3-year follow-up. Good to excellent clinical results were seen in 11 of 12 patients (91.6%).[41] Subjective outcomes, as measured by the physical component of the SF-36 survey, averaged more than 90 points. Average time to return to full athletic participation was 3.7 months. Single incision techniques have shown slightly lower success rates than dual incision.[42] Female athletes may respond less favorably to fasciotomy and have shown lower success rates with surgery when compared with male athletes.[43]

COMPLICATIONS

Reported complications of surgical treatment include hematoma or seroma formation, wound infection, peripheral nerve injury, and deep venous thrombosis. Incidence of postoperative complications ranges from 2% to 13%.[14,32,37,38] Targeting the reduction of hematoma can be performed by controlling all bleeders at the time of surgery, avoiding the use of a tourniquet at the time of surgery, and postoperative compression dressings with cryotherapy. Reducing the risk of cellulites and infection can be accomplished with careful tissue handling at the time of surgery, antibiotic irrigation at the time of wound closures, perioperative antibiotics for 3 days, and aggressive control of postoperative swelling and hematoma. Avoiding or reducing the risk of nerve injury is accomplished by carefully identifying the superficial peroneal nerve and protecting it during the fascial release. Avoiding or preventing postoperative deep venous thrombosis can be accomplished via early postoperative mobilization and screening for at-risk patients. We routinely use aspirin for 2 to 3 weeks postoperatively and reserve formal anticoagulation therapy for patients with known risk factors. Nonetheless, it must be acknowledged that a more formal approach of routine anticoagulation therapy would also be reasonable but would likely increase the risk of postoperative hematoma.

Recurrence of symptoms has been reported in 2% to 17% of patients after fasciotomy.[32,38] Recurrence may be caused by incomplete release of an affected compartment, failure to release all affected compartments, or fascial scarring during healing after fasciotomy. In a porcine study in our laboratory, we were able to determine that an 80% release of the fascia was adequate for a 100% decompression of the intracompartmental pressures. Revision surgery may be necessary in patients with recurrent symptoms.

SUMMARY

Chronic exertional compartment syndrome is a relatively common, but often overlooked cause of leg pain in athletes. A careful history and physical examination is essential in the diagnosis of CECS. Affected individuals have recurrent, activity-related leg pain that recurs at a consistent duration or intensity and is only relieved by rest. Measurement of baseline and postexercise compartment pressures confirms the diagnosis and helps in the planning of treatment. Surgical treatment with fasciotomy of the involved compartments is successful in allowing patients to return to full activity levels. With surgical treatment, it is critical to address all affected compartments as well as releasing any fascial defects, both of which may cause recurrent symptoms if neglected. With appropriate diagnosis and treatment, excellent outcomes can be achieved and allow athletes to return to full, unrestricted activity levels.

REFERENCES

1. Clanton TO, Solcher BW. Chronic leg pain in the athlete. Clin Sports Med 1994;13(4): 743–59.

2. Styf J. Diagnosis of exercise-induced pain in the anterior aspect of the lower leg. Am J Sports Med 1988;16(2):165–9.

3. Edmundsson D, Toolanen G, Sojka P. Chronic compartment syndrome also affects nonathletic subjects: a prospective study of 63 cases with exercise-induced lower leg pain. Acta Orthop 2007;78(1):136–42.

4. Edmundsson D, Toolanen G. Chronic exertional compartment syndrome in diabetes mellitus. Diabet Med 2011;28(1):81–5.

5. Mavor GE. The anterior tibial syndrome. J Bone Joint Surg Br 1956;38–B(2):513–7.

6. Kirby NG. Exercise ischaemia in the fascial compartment of soleus. Report of a case. J Bone Joint Surg Br 1970;52(4):738–40.

7. Puranen J. The medial tibial syndrome: exercise ischaemia in the medial fascial compartment of the leg. J Bone Joint Surg Br 1974;56–B(4):712–5.

8. Edwards P, Myerson MS. Exertional compartment syndrome of the leg: steps for expedient return to activity. Phys Sportsmed 1996;24(4):31–46.

9. Lundvall J, Mellander S, Westling H, et al. Fluid transfer between blood and tissues during exercise. Acta Physiol Scand 1972;85(2):258–69.

10. Fronek J, Mubarak SJ, Hargens AR, et al. Management of chronic exertional anterior compartment syndrome of the lower extremity. Clin Orthop Relat Res 1987;(220):217–27.

11. Reneman RS. The anterior and the lateral compartmental syndrome of the leg due to intensive use of muscles. Clin Orthop Relat Res 1975;(113):69–80.

12. Edmundsson D, Toolanen G, Thornell LE, et al. Evidence for low muscle capillary supply as a pathogenic factor in chronic compartment syndrome. Scand J Med Sci Sports 2010;20(6):805–13.

13. Jones DC, James SL. Overuse injuries of the lower extremity: shin splints, iliotibial band friction syndrome, and exertional compartment syndromes. Clin Sports Med 1987;6(2):273–90.

14. Detmer DE, Sharpe K, Sufit RL, et al. Chronic compartment syndrome: diagnosis, management, and outcomes. Am J Sports Med 1985;13(3):162–70.

15. Whitesides TE Jr, Haney TC, Harada H, et al. A simple method for tissue pressure determination. Arch Surg 1975;110(11):1311–3.

16. Rorabeck CH, Castle GS, Hardie R, et al. Compartmental pressure measurements: an experimental investigation using the slit catheter. J Trauma 1981;21(6):446–9.

17. McDermott AG, Marble AE, Yabsley RH, et al. Monitoring dynamic anterior compartment pressures during exercise. A new technique using the STIC catheter. Am J Sports Med 1982;10(2):83–9.

18. Mubarak SJ, Hargens AR, Owen CA, et al. The wick catheter technique for measurement of intramuscular pressure. A new research and clinical tool. J Bone Joint Surg Am 1976;58(7):1016–20.

19. Styf JR, Korner LM. Microcapillary infusion technique for measurement of intramuscular pressure during exercise. Clin Orthop Relat Res 1986;(207):253–62.

20. Glorioso J, Wilckens J. Compartment syndrome testing. In: O'Connor F, Wilder R, editors. The textbook of running medicine. New York: McGraw-Hill; 2001. p. 95–100.

21. Pedowitz RA, Hargens AR, Mubarak SJ, et al. Modified criteria for the objective diagnosis of chronic compartment syndrome of the leg. Am J Sports Med 1990;18(1):35–40.

22. Whitesides TE, Heckman MM. Acute compartment syndrome: update on diagnosis and treatment. J Am Acad Orthop Surg 1996;4(4):209–18.

23. Hislop M, Batt ME. Chronic exertional compartment syndrome. Br J Sports Med 2011;45(12):954–5.

24. Hutchinson M. Chronic exertional compartment syndrome head to head. Br J Sports Med 2011. [Epub ahead of print].

25. Wiley JP, Short WB, Wiseman DA, et al. Ultrasound catheter placement for deep posterior compartment pressure measurements in chronic compartment syndrome. Am J Sports Med 1990;18(1):74–9.

26. Peck E, Finnoff JT, Smith J, et al. Accuracy of palpation-guided and ultrasound-guided needle tip placement into the deep and superficial posterior leg compartments. Am J Sports Med 2011;39(9):1968–74.

27. Mohler LR, Styf JR, Pedowitz RA, et al. Intramuscular deoxygenation during exercise in patients who have chronic anterior compartment syndrome of the leg. J Bone Joint Surg Am 1997;79(6):844–9.

28. Breit GA, Gross JH, Watenpaugh DE, et al. Near-infrared spectroscopy for monitoring of tissue oxygenation of exercising skeletal muscle in a chronic compartment syndrome model. J Bone Joint Surg Am 1997;79(6):838–43.

29. Verleisdonk EJ, van Gils A, van der Werken C. The diagnostic value of MRI scans for the diagnosis of chronic exertional compartment syndrome of the lower leg. Skeletal Radiol 2001;30(6):321–5.

30. Amendola A, Rorabeck CH, Vellett D, et al. The use of magnetic resonance imaging in exertional compartment syndromes. Am J Sports Med 1990;18(1):29–34.

31. Takebayashi S, Takazawa H, Sasaki R, et al. Chronic exertional compartment syndrome in lower legs: localization and follow-up with thallium-201 SPECT imaging. J Nucl Med 1997;38(6):972–6.

32. Rorabeck CH, Fowler PJ, Nott L. The results of fasciotomy in the management of chronic exertional compartment syndrome. Am J Sports Med 1988;16(3):224–7.

33. Styf JR, Korner LM. Chronic anterior-compartment syndrome of the leg. Results of treatment by fasciotomy. J Bone Joint Surg Am 1986;68(9):1338–47.

34. Wood ML, Almekinders LC. Minimally invasive subcutaneous fasciotomy for chronic exertional compartment syndrome of the lower extremity. Am J Orthop (Belle Mead NJ). 2004;33(1):42–4.

35. Leversedge FJ, Casey PJ, Seiler JG 3rd, et al. Endoscopically assisted fasciotomy: description of technique and in vitro assessment of lower-leg compartment decompression. Am J Sports Med 2002;30(2):272–8.

36. Wittstein J, Moorman CT 3rd, Levin LS. Endoscopic compartment release for chronic exertional compartment syndrome: surgical technique and results. Am J Sports Med 2010;38(8):1661–6.

37. Hutchinson MR, Bederka B, Kopplin M. Anatomic structures at risk during minimal-incision endoscopically assisted fascial compartment releases in the leg. Am J Sports Med 2003;31(5):764–9.

38. Schepsis AA, Martini D, Corbett M. Surgical management of exertional compartment syndrome of the lower leg. Long-term followup. Am J Sports Med 1993;21(6):811–7[discussion: 817].

39. Schubert AG. Exertional compartment syndrome: review of the literature and proposed rehabilitation guidelines following surgical release. Int J Sports Phys Ther 2011;6(2):126–41.

40. Howard JL, Mohtadi NG, Wiley JP. Evaluation of outcomes in patients following surgical treatment of chronic exertional compartment syndrome in the leg. Clin J Sport Med 2000;10(3):176–84.

41. Meinenger A, Hutchinson M, editors. Athletes with chronic exertional compartment syndrome: results of two-incision endoscopic assisted fasciotomy at 3 years. Amelia Island (FL): Mid-America Orthopaedic Association; 2009.

42. Slimmon D, Bennell K, Brukner P, et al. Long-term outcome of fasciotomy with partial fasciectomy for chronic exertional compartment syndrome of the lower leg. Am J Sports Med 2002;30(4):581–8.
43. Micheli LJ, Solomon R, Solomon J, et al. Surgical treatment for chronic lower-leg compartment syndrome in young female athletes. Am J Sports Med 1999;27(2):197–201.

Popliteal Entrapment in Runners

William D. Turnipseed, MD

KEYWORDS

- Runners leg pain • Popliteal entrapment
- Compartment syndrome

Popliteal entrapment syndrome, a term originally coined by Love and Whelan in 1965,[1] is a rare form of overuse injury clinically manifest by a complex of neuromuscular or ischemia symptoms in the lower extremity resulting from pathologic impingement behind the knee. In 1879, Stuart[2] documented an apparent relationship between popliteal artery occlusion, ischemic gangrene, and an abnormal passage of the popliteal artery medially around the medial head of the gastrocnemius muscle. Since then, numerous congenital variations in the development and insertion of the gastrocnemius and popliteus muscles have been documented as a cause for pathologic impingement behind the knee.[3,4] Vascular anomalies, such as aberrant geniculate branches, have also been described as unusual sources for impingement.[5] These abnormalities, although quite rare, are associated with an increased risk of threatening lower extremity ischemia, particularly in adolescents and young adults. Focal impingement results in repetitive microtrauma to the popliteal vessels, causing chronic inflammation and subsequent occlusive or aneurysmal change. These vascular anomalies are responsible for embolic and thrombotic events that result in claudication or limb-threatening ischemia.

Popliteal entrapment syndrome associated with aberrant musculotendinous impingement requires surgical intervention. Saphenous vein bypass is the most commonly performed procedure when arterial stenosis, occlusion, or aneurysm is present. If there is no significant intrinsic vascular disease associated with impingement, the retrogeniculate approach is appropriate, with resection of the offending muscle band or ligation and transection of the aberrant geniculate vessels causing impingement.[6]

The anatomic form of popliteal entrapment should always be suspected when isolated lower extremity ischemia (claudication, embolism) occurs in young adults with no evidence of cardiac or diffuse peripheral vascular disease.

In 1985, a French surgeon named Rignault described an atypical form of claudication in military recruits.[7] He documented lateral arterial impingement with stress positional

The author has nothing to disclose.

Division of Vascular Surgery, Department of Surgery, University of Wisconsin School of Medicine and Public Health, 600 Highland Avenue, G5/325, Madison, WI 53792, USA

E-mail address: turnip@surgery.wisc.edu

Clin Sports Med 31 (2012) 321–328

doi:10.1016/j.csm.2011.09.010

sportsmed.theclinics.com

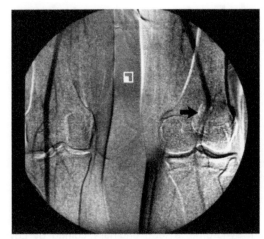

Fig. 1. Digital subtraction arteriogram study shows lateral displacement of the popliteal artery in neutral position (*right*), and long segment occlusion with plantar flexion (*left*) characteristic of functional impingement. (*Courtesy of* W. D. Turnipseed, MD, Madison, WI.)

arteriography and operated expecting to find aberrant muscle compression. The only significant finding was a hypertrophic medial belly of the gastrocnemius muscle. He subsequently referred to this condition as the functional popliteal entrapment syndrome.[7] A few years later, we encountered a number of track and cross country athletes that complained of atypical symptoms described by Rignault. These included deep upper calf muscle cramping made worse when running on inclines or repetitive jumping and occasional plantar paresthesias. We did stress positional magnetic resonance imaging (MRI)/magnetic resonance angiography (MRA) studies and found that there was long segmental lateral compression of the neurovascular bundle. Proximal compression resulted from contraction of a hypertrophic medial gastrocnemius and plantaris muscle forcing the neurovascular bundle against the lateral condyle of the femur. Distally, with plantar flexion, the soleus muscle compressed the vascular bundle against the lateral soleal band forming the outlet of the popliteal fossa (**Figs. 1** and **2**).[8]

The exact cause for symptoms in patients with functional popliteal entrapment is not clearly understood.[9] Although ischemic symptoms have been documented in elderly patients with functional impingement, we have not documented any arterial complications in adolescents or young adults. Our impression is that the symptoms result from nerve compression against the lateral soleal fascia that forms a narrowed exit from the popliteal fossa.[8]

PATIENT WORKUP

All patients suspected of having popliteal entrapment syndrome have a detailed history, physical examination, and selective noninvasive vascular testing. All patients had ankle brachial indices and stress positional plethysmography using the Pulse Volume Recorder (Parks Medical Electronics, Inc, Aloha, OR, USA) to screen for arterial occlusive disorders and for popliteal entrapment. Duplex vascular imaging was commonly used to evaluate patients that presented with chronic limb swelling or positional limb swelling to rule out postphlebitic syndrome, venous valvular incompetence, or venous popliteal entrapment.[10] Duplex studies were also performed in

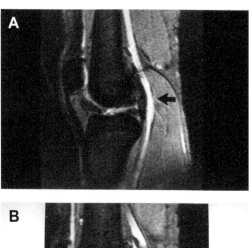

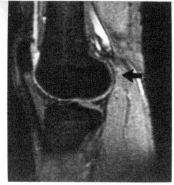

Fig. 2. MRA shows impingement of the popliteal artery by medial head of the gastrocnemius muscle with plantar flexion. (*A*) Neutral position. (*B*) Plantar flexion. (*Courtesy of* W. D. Turnipseed, MD, Madison, WI.)

those patients who had a palpable mass behind the knee to rule out popliteal aneurysm or a Baker's cyst. Occasionally, 3-phase nuclear bone scanning was performed in patients with chronic medial tibial bone pain to rule out the presence of periostitis or microcortical tibial fracture.

Popliteal entrapment screening was done with stress positional testing using a 10-cm cuff inflated to 60 mm Hg with the patient in supine position, knees extended and the foot in neutral, forced plantar and dorsi flexion positions. Abnormal stress positional tests consisted of an ankle brachial index drop rate greater than 30% or flattening of plethysmographic waveforms in plantar or dorsi flexion or both (**Fig. 3**). We don't routinely use stress positional duplex imaging unless we suspect venous impingement may be associated with popliteal entrapment. We find that stress positional plethysmography is cheaper and less time consuming than duplex imaging, and we have not documented that plethysmography or duplex imaging by themselves are helpful in determining whether abnormal musculotendinous structures are responsible for popliteal impingement.[5]

Although digital contrast for MRA is appropriate for evaluating patients with suspected intrinsic arterial disease, we have found that the combination of stress positional T2-weighted MRI and MRA are preferred for the evaluation of patients that are suspected of having popliteal entrapment. This combination of studies allows for definition of normal and abnormal musculotendinous structures within the popliteal

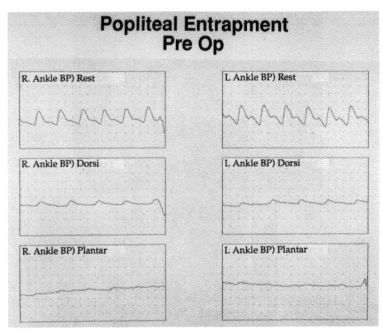

Fig. 3. The positional plethysmographic screening test shows vascular impingement with plantar flexion of the feet. (*Courtesy of* W. D. Turnipseed, MD, Madison, WI.)

fossa as well as for providing accurate arterial imaging in younger healthy patients.[11,12]

We routinely perform compartment pressure measurements when symptoms are associated with the upper posterior calf muscles. Resting pressures are measured bilaterally even if the complaints are unilateral. Pressures after exercise were only performed if patients have been inactive for more than a month before the examination because a prolonged period of inactivity results in a loss of muscle tone and compartment pressures that don't accurately reflect the active conditioning of the athlete. When exercise testing is required, we have the patient run outside the clinic until symptoms develop and return for pressure measurements. We do this because the time required to develop complaints often is prolonged, and the conditions on the treadmill don't accurately reflect the running environment for most training athletes. Normally, postexercise pressures return to baseline within 3 to 5 minutes. With this in mind, we usually wait 10 minutes and then measure pressures to rule out the presence of a posterior superficial compartment syndrome.[13]

RESULTS

We have surgically treated nearly 1700 patients for atypical claudication associated with popliteal entrapment or chronic recurrent compartment syndromes (CRECS). A total of 2500 fasciectomies have been performed for CRECS (anterior lateral 47%, posterior superficial 44%, deep posterior 9%), and 68 popliteal entrapment releases (51 Functional Popliteal Artery Entrapment Syndrome (FPAES) releases [75%], 17 anatomic releases [25%]) in this cohort of adolescents and young adults. The FPAES patients were typically young athletic women (mean age, 26 years) with no evidence

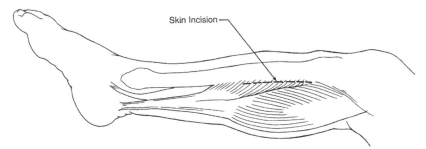

Skin Incision

Fig. 4. Functional entrapment release is performed through a medial calf incision similar to that used to expose the popliteal artery for distal bypass. It is important to avoid injury to the saphenous vein or nerve. The first element of the release procedure is excision of the fascia overlying the gastrocnemius and soleus muscles. (*Courtesy of* W. D. Turnipseed, MD, Madison, WI.)

of ischemia and isolated symptoms of soleus muscle cramping and plantar paresthesias. Two presented with intermittent calf swelling and popliteal vein impingement. Nearly half of the FPAES patients either had coexistent symptoms of CRECS or had been surgically treated for CRECS before entrapment release. The anatomic entrapment patients were predominantly men (70%), mean age 46 years, with ischemic symptoms of claudication or digital embolization. One patient had a popliteal aneurysm and the rest had popliteal artery stenosis or occlusion. When arterial repair is indicated, we use the retrogeniculate approach and preferentially use endarterectomy or arterial resection and reanastomosis in these young patients with diseased but patent arteries. Vein bypass is required for arterial occlusions.[12] We do not favor endovascular stent placement or angioplasty as a primary treatment for anatomic entrapment because the mechanism for arterial injury remains, and early recurrence has been documented in the literature.[14]

Different surgical procedures have been proposed for the treatment of FPAES. A posterior approach with myectomy of the medial head of the gastroc muscle leaving the tendinous insertion has been proposed and shown to be successful in relieving symptoms.[15] We prefer a medial calf approach through an incision similar to that used for accessing the tibial peroneal trunk of the popliteal artery when doing a distal bypass (**Fig. 4**). Our belief is that the major problem occurs not proximally but distally at the exit of the popliteal fossa and feel that taking down the soleal fascia band has provided relief and does not affect muscle function, particularly in highly trained athletes (**Fig. 5**).[16]

DISCUSSION

Popliteal entrapment syndromes have generated considerable interests in the surgical community because they have been associated with disabling symptoms and the potential for serious morbidity in young otherwise healthy individuals with active lifestyles.[17,18] As noninvasive screening techniques such as duplex, computed tomography, or MRI have become more widely utilized in the evaluation of patients with lower extremity claudication, detection of popliteal impingement has become more frequent. Current literature suggests that impingement of neurovascular structures behind the knee is, in fact, quite common in young adults and may occur in 50% to 80% of otherwise asymptomatic age-controlled study groups.[19–21] Furthermore, there appears to be a significant difference in clinic presentation and morbidity risk in

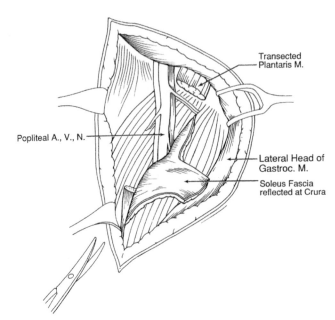

Transected Plantaris M.

Popliteal A., V., N.

Lateral Head of Gastroc. M.

Soleus Fascia reflected at Crura

Fig. 5. The functional entrapment release is completed by resecting the plantaris muscle (which is frequently hypertrophic) and then resecting the crural band of soleus fascia that forms the outlet of the popliteal fossa. This fascial band is the fulcrum against which the neurovascular bundle is compressed. (*Courtesy of* W. D. Turnipseed, MD, Madison, WI.)

symptomatic patients with documented popliteal vascular compression based on the presence or absence of aberrant musculotendinous structures behind the knee. Although a clear relationship exists between the development of local occlusive or aneurysmal changes in the popliteal artery of patients with impingement caused by musculotendinous anomalies in the popliteal fossa, the prevalence and natural history of popliteal impingement is less certain when it occurs in the absence of any anatomic abnormality. Symptomatic functional popliteal impingement seems much more common in athletically active young adults and is rarely associated with intrinsic vascular change or ischemic morbidity. Although the exact cause for claudication symptoms remains uncertain in these patients, we think nerve compression within the soleal canal is the most likely explanation, much like the neuromuscular complaints associated with thoracic outlet syndrome.

Surgeons should understand that the prognosis and cause for symptoms differ in patients with anatomic and functional forms of impingement, and they should be aware of demographic differences between the 2 groups. Patients with anatomic entrapment are commonly male (70%), older (mean age 43 years), more sedentary, and have restrictive claudication symptoms (exercise distance less than two blocks) associated with focal popliteal artery disease. Patients with functional entrapment are younger (mean age 24 years) and more commonly female (70%) who are well conditioned athletes or have active lifestyles. Functional popliteal entrapment syndrome appears to be a form of overuse injury and is more likely to occur in the same population afflicted with chronic compartment syndromes. This is reflected by the fact that more than 30% of all patients we have treated for chronic compartment syndrome have positive popliteal impingement screening studies, yet less than 12% ever have symptoms referable to these findings.

The fact that chronic compartment syndrome and functional popliteal entrapment syndrome tend to occur in the same cohort of patients creates a diagnostic dilemma creating the necessity for correct diagnosis in patients with posterior calf complaints to offer appropriate treatment. In our experience, chronic compartment syndrome is much more common than symptomatic functional popliteal entrapment. With this in mind, it is important to rule out symptomatic chronic compartment syndrome in patients that present with atypical claudication manifest by upper posterior calf pain and plantar paresthesia. FPAES and CRECS are frequently confused with one another because the complaints are similar in quality and anatomic location and often overlap.[16]

We have found that symptomatic popliteal entrapment syndrome is a very uncommon cause for atypical claudication symptoms. The functional form of popliteal impingement associated with symptoms is much more common than the anatomic form of popliteal entrapment. We recommend that young patients with calf claudication and no obvious orthopedic or vascular risk factors should have noninvasive testing, such as stress plethysmography or duplex imaging, to rule out popliteal entrapment syndrome. Symptomatic patients with positive noninvasive impingement studies should have peripheral vascular imaging with stress positional arteriography. We prefer the use of stress positional MRI/MRA because it affords a risk-free opportunity to evaluate musculoskeletal structures in the popliteal fossa as well as vascular anatomy. Because of the discrepancy between the prevalence of popliteal impingement and the actual development of symptoms, we feel that prophylactic surgical correction of functional impingement in asymptomatic patients is inappropriate. However, surgical treatment for symptomatic forms of anatomic treatment make sense as does the prophylactic treatment of asymptomatic contralateral disease because of the established risk for vascular morbidity.

It is important for surgeons to establish the correct diagnosis to afford the patient a high probability of treatment cure. Adolescents and young adults with atypical forms of claudication that develop in the absence of musculoskeletal injury or vascular risk factors may suffer from popliteal entrapment or chronic compartment syndromes. Noninvasive stress positional testing can screen for impingement; however, these tests are not capable of distinguishing functional from anatomic forms of the disease. Stress positional imaging and soft tissue assessment looking for musculotendinous anomalies behind the knee are critically important to plan appropriate surgical care. In patients with appropriate symptoms and vascular imaging studies suggesting functional popliteal entrapment, posterior superficial compartment pressures measurements are essential to distinguish chronic compartment syndrome from the functional entrapment disorder.

REFERENCES

1. Love JW, Whelan TJ. Popliteal artery entrapment syndrome. Am J Surg 1965;109: 620–4.
2. Stuart TP. Note on a variation in the course of the popliteal artery. J Anat Physiol 1879;13:162.
3. Insua JA, Young JR, Humphries AW. Popliteal artery entrapment syndrome. Arch Surg 1970;101:771–5.
4. Rich NM, Hughes CW. Popliteal artery and vein entrapment. Am J Surg 1967;113: 696–8.
5. Turnipseed WD. Popliteal entrapment syndrome. J Vasc Surg 2002;35:910–5.

6. di Marzo L, Cavallaro A, Sciacca V, et al. Surgical treatment of popliteal artery entrapment syndrome: a ten year experience. Eur J Vasc Surg 1991;51:518–22.

7. Rignault DP, Pailler JL, Lunel F. The 'functional' popliteal entrapment syndrome. Int Angiol 1985;4:341–3.

8. Turnipseed WD, Pozniak M. Popliteal entrapment as a result of neurovascular compression by the soleus and plantaris muscles. J Vasc Surg 1992;15:285–94.

9. Levien LJ, Veller MG. Popliteal artery entrapment syndrome: more common than previously recognized. J Vasc Surg 1999;30:587–98.

10. di Marzo L, Cavallaro A, Sciacca V, et al. Diagnosis of popliteal artery entrapment syndrome: the role of duplex scanning. J Vasc Surg 1991;13:434–8.

11. Stager A, Clement D. Popliteal artery entrapment syndrome. Sports Med 1999;28:61–70.

12. Turnipseed WD. Clinical review of patients treated for atypical claudication: a 28-year experience. J Vasc Surg 2004;40:79–85.

13. Turnipseed WD. Atypical claudication associated with overuse injury in patients with chronic compartment, functional entrapment, and medical tibial stress syndromes. Cardiovascular Surgery 2003;11:421–3.

14. di Marzo L, Cavallaro A, O'Donnell SD, et al. Endovascular stenting for popliteal vascular entrapment is not recommended. Ann Vasc Surg 2010;24:1135,e1–1135,e3.

15. Causey MW, Singh N, Miller S, et al. Intraoperative duplex and functional popliteal entrapment syndrome: strategy for effective treatment. Ann Vasc Surg 2010;24:556–61.

16. Turnipseed WD. Functional popliteal artery entrapment syndrome: a poorly understood and often missed diagnosis that is frequently mistreated. J Vasc Surg 2009;49:1189–95.

17. Boskamp M, Ijpma FF, Meerwalkdt R, et al. Serious morbidity associated with popliteal artery entrapment syndrome. Clin J Sport Med 2009;19:435–7.

18. Housseini AM, Maged IM, Abdel-Gawad EA, et al. Popliteal artery entrapment syndrome. J Vasc Surg 2009;49:1056.

19. Erdoes LS, Devine JJ, Vernhard VM, et al. Popliteal vascular compression in a normal population. J Vasc Surg 1994;20:978–86.

20. Pillai J, Levien LJ, Haagensen M, et al. Assessment of the medial head of the gastrocnemius muscle in functional compression of the popliteal artery. J Vasc Surg 2008;48:1189–96.

21. Pillai J. A current interpretation of popliteal vascular entrapment. J Vasc Surg 2008;48:61S–65S.

Tendinopathy Treatment: Where is the Evidence?

Christian C. Skjong, MD[a], Alexander K. Meininger, MD[b],*,
Sherwin S.W. Ho, MD[a]

KEYWORDS

• Tendinopathy • Tendinitis • Overuse injury • Running athlete

Overuse syndromes are the most common injuries in runners. Up to 70% of runners experience overuse injuries in a 1-year period with such diagnoses as tendinosis, "shin splints," stress fractures or fasciitis.[1] Although 75% of these injuries are below the knee,[2] patellar, Achilles, and peroneal tendinopathy rank among the most common overuse conditions in the running athlete.[3]

PREVALENCE

In epidemiologic terms, overuse injuries, including tendinopathy, account for approximately 7% of all physician office visits in the United States.[4,5] This is in large part because of the increased participation in recreational sports as well as the increased duration and intensity of training within organized athletics.[6] In fact, greater than 30% of injuries related to sports activity result from or have a component of tendinopathy.[7] More specifically, 30% of all running-related injuries and 40% of all elbow injuries in tennis players are the direct result of tendinopathy.[8] The prevalence of patellar tendinopathy is as high as 32% and 45% in basketball and volleyball players, respectively.[8] Interestingly, tendinopathy is not only an affliction of the physically active. Although Achilles tendinopathy is traditionally seen in association with running and jumping activities, a significant percentage of cases have been found in those leading a sedentary lifestyle.[9–11]

Given the widespread prevalence and incidence of tendinopathy in the general public, much effort has been placed in determining the most beneficial and

Dr Skjong and Dr Meininger have no disclosures.
Disclosures: Biomet (Consultant, speaker), Smith and Nephew (Fellowship Grant, speaker), OREF (Fellowship Grant), Omega Medical Grants Association (Fellowship Grant), AANA (multiple committees), AOSSM (Council of Delegates), IAOS (Past President, Board of Directors), Medscape Reference/WebMD (Editor In Chief, Sports Medicine).
[a] Department of Surgery, Section of Orthopaedics and Rehabilitation, University of Chicago Hospital, 5841 South Maryland, M/C 3079, Chicago, IL 60637, USA
[b] Orthopaedic Surgery & Sports Medicine, Moab Regional Specialty Clinic, 476 West Williams Way, Suite B, Moab, UT 84532, USA
* Corresponding author.
E-mail address: DrAlex@mrhmoab.org

cost-effective treatments available. The goal of this review was to provide a comprehensive and up-to-date analysis of treatment options, including eccentric exercises, injection therapies, extracorporeal shockwave therapy, and operative management.

PATHOPHYSIOLOGY

Tendinopathy is a general descriptor that includes any painful condition occurring within or around a tendon. Often in response to overuse, it is characterized by activity-related pain, focal tenderness to palpation, and decreased strength in the affected area. Tendinopathy is often labeled an overuse injury theoretically resulting from tendon cells being exposed to a high volume of repetitive load. Certain anatomic locations are therefore predisposed to injury, including the Achilles, peroneal, posterior tibial, hamstring, patella, and various upper extremity tendons. For example, the Achilles tendon is one of the more common entities affected. This is not surprising, as the Achilles bears stresses of up to 12.5 times that of normal body weight during ambulation and even greater during strenuous physical activity.[8] Tendon tissue is specifically designed to handle this chronic stress. Oxygen consumption has been shown to be 7.5 times lower in tendons than in skeletal muscle.[9] This low metabolic rate and anaerobic energy-generating capacity is essential to allow the tendon to maintain tension and carry loads for prolonged periods. The tradeoff to this evolutionary advantage, however, is a slower rate of healing after injury, an element that certainly contributes to the chronicity of pain seen in cases of tendinopathy.

For many years, the term *tendonitis* was used to describe these conditions, implying a component of inflammation contributed to the underlying pathology. Recent basic science research, however, has refuted this claim. Histologic analysis of tendinopathic tissue has found very little evidence of inflammatory cell involvement in affected tendons (**Fig. 1**).[1,2] Instead, marked disorganization within the collagen bundles is seen compared with normal tendon (**Table 1**).[2–4] Affected tendon also shows an increased infiltration of new blood vessels and nerves. This neovascularization is thought to contribute to the pain symptoms commonly associated with tendinopathy.[3,5–7] These pathologic changes are more accurately described as a cycle of degeneration and attempted regeneration than to an inflammatory process.

PHARMACOTHERAPY
Anti-inflammatories

Traditionally, nonsteroidal anti-inflammatory drugs (NSAIDs) have been used as a treatment for tendon overuse injuries for decades. Classically, and most commonly, oral administration has been the preferred application; although, local NSAID administration, through the use of gels or patches, has recently become an acceptable alternative. There are, however, 2 flaws with this approach. First, there is little histologic or biochemical evidence of inflammation in the pathogenesis of tendinopathy.[12] In fact, anti-inflammatories may actually inhibit tendon healing in response to injury.[13] Secondly, limited quality evidence exists to support the use of NSAIDs for pain associated with chronic overuse tendon injuries.

Although there has been significant investigation into the efficacy of NSAIDs in the treatment of tendinopathy, contradictory data exists. For instance, a randomized, double-blind, placebo-controlled trial failed to find any clinical benefit of piroxicam to placebo in Achilles tendinopathy.[14] Overall, evidence supports their use in both oral and local forms with clear benefits as short-term analgesics (7–14 days).[15–21] There is unfortunately little evidence showing a benefit to long-term symptomatic reprieve. A study by Hay and colleagues[20] looking at cases of lateral epicondylitis, for example,

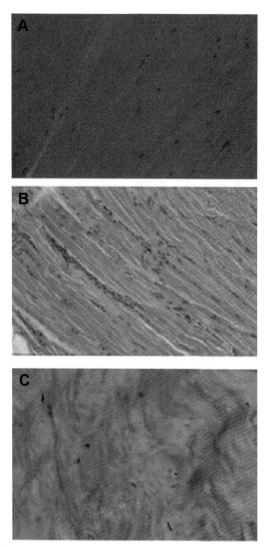

Fig. 1. Histopathologic changes seen in tendinopathy show a lack of an inflammatory response. (*A*) Normal tendon with scattered elongated cells. (*B*) Slightly pathologic tendinous tissue with islands of high cellularity and initial disorganization. (*C*) Highly degenerated tendon with some chondroid cells; there is a distinct lack of inflammatory infiltrate. (*From* Rees JD, Maffulli N, Cook J. Management of tendinopathy. Am J Sports Med 2009;37(9):1856; with permission.)

reported no significant difference between naproxen sodium and placebo at 1-year follow-up.

In general, a short course of NSAIDs appears to be an effective first-line treatment for acute pain relief associated with tendinopathy. It is important to remember, however, that these medications carry a risk of gastrointestinal, cardiovascular, and renal complications and should not be used for chronic treatment of symptoms.

Table 1
Comparison of normal and tendinopathic tendon

Findings	Macroscopic	Grey-scale or Color and Power Doppler Ultrasound Scan	Light Microscopic
Normal Tendon	Brilliant white Fibroelastic firm texture	Parallel hyperechoic or bright white line Regular uniform fiber structure	Organized parallel collagen bundles Spindle shape tenocyte nuclei Nuclei parallel alignment
Tendinopathy Tendon	Grey or brown Tissue is thin, fragile and disorganized Loose texture	Localized widening of the tendon Local hypoechoic areas Irregular fiber structure Neovascularization correlated with tendon changes	Disorganized collagen bundle Increased ground substance consisting of proteoglycans and glycosaminoglycans Large mucoid patches and vacuoles between fibers Round with darker-staining tenocyte nuclei Markedly increased number of nuclei with loss of parallel alignment Increase of vascular and nerve ingrowths Densely packed collagen fibers Uniform in diameter and orientation of collagen fibers Angulation, bubble formation of collagen fibers Variations in the diameters and orientation of collagen fibers Hyperoxic changes in tenocytes (lipid vacuoles, enlarged lysosomes and degranulated endoplasmic retinaculum

From Xu Y, Murrell GAC. The basic science of tendinopathy. Clin Orthop Relat Res 2008;466(7):1528–38; with permission.

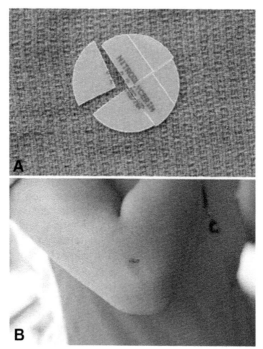

Fig. 2. (A) Prescription 5-mg/24-hour nitroglycerin patches are cut into quarters and (B) and placed directly over the point of maximal tenderness. (*From* Andres BM, Murrell GA. Treatment of tendinopathy: what works, what doesn't and what's on the horizon. Clin Orthop Relat Res 2008;466:1541; with permission.)

Glycerol Trinitrate

Topical glycerol trinitrate (GTN) has been investigated by the US Food and Drug Administration for off-label use in the treatment of tendinopathy. Nitroglycerin patches are divided into quarters and applied to the point of maximal tenderness (**Fig. 2**). Topical nitroglycerin, or GTN, is a prodrug of endogenous nitric oxide, more commonly known for its use in angina pectoris. Nitric acid synthase converts GTN into bioactive nitric oxide molecules. Nitric oxide has been shown to induce fibroblast proliferation and collagen synthesis in a rat Achilles tendon model.[22] Furthermore, nitric oxide synthase inhibition results in decreased cross-sectional area and load to failure in healing tendon.[23]

Seven randomized, controlled trials performed outside the United States have evaluated the effectiveness of topical GTN in the treatment of tendinopathy.[21,24-28] A recent meta-analysis (including these studies) concluded that topical GTN provides symptomatic relief for tendinopathy.[29] The most common side effect across all studies was headache. One trial examining 58 patients with lateral epicondylitis showed a clinical benefit of GTN over tendon rehabilitation alone at 24 weeks with improved pain, resumption of activities of daily living, and overall outcomes.[21] However, a follow-up study including 70% of the same patients 5-years after cessation of treatment showed no long-term clinical benefit.[30] Thus far, data clearly show GTN provides short-term pain relief in tendinopathy sufferers; although long-term benefit remains in question.

ECCENTRIC EXERCISE

Eccentric exercise has long been utilized as a component in rehabilitation and treatment of various forms of tendinopathy. Eccentric muscle contractions are those in which a muscle elongates while under tension (**Fig. 3**). Compared with concentric exercises (muscle fibers contract under tension), eccentric movements result in less oxygen consumption, less energy expenditure, and greater force production.[31] It is hypothesized that this creates an environment with less heat and fewer waste products generated, thereby reducing irritative variables that could hamper tendon healing.

A large body of evidence exists promoting the efficacy of eccentric training in the treatment of tendinopathy. Shalabi and colleagues[32] evaluated 25 patients with chronic Achilles tendinopathy with magnetic resonance imaging before and after an eccentric exercise program. Their results showed decreased tendon volume and intratendinous signal intensity, which correlated with decreased pain and improved performance.[32] A histologic study performed by Langberg and coworkers[33] found increases in type 1 collagen in cases of Achilles tendinopathy after an eccentric exercise program, indicating the direct effect of physiotherapy on the healing of injured tendon.

Clinical studies focusing solely on patient outcomes, such as pain and return to sport, have exhibited significant improvements in patients receiving eccentric exercise treatment compared with other modalities, such as concentric exercises or observation alone.[33-39] Silbernagel and coworkers[40] recently reported on patients with Achilles tendinopathy treated solely with physical therapy incorporating eccentric exercises. Five-year follow-up found 80% of patients fully recovered with complete pain relief.[40] Synergistic effects have also been found when eccentric exercises are included in a multidisciplinary treatment algorithm. A recent randomized, controlled trial[41] including cases of Achilles tendinopathy found that eccentric exercise in combination with low energy shock-wave therapy resulted in even more improvement in patient-measured outcomes when compared with eccentric exercises alone, highlighting the potential benefits of combined treatment regimens.

In general, eccentric exercise is an accessible and effective treatment of tendinopathy with no reported adverse effects and should strongly be considered as a first-line intervention.

EXTRACORPOREAL SHOCK WAVE THERAPY

Extracorporeal shockwave therapy (ESWT) has been used for treatment of various soft tissue injuries, including tendinopathy. ESWT involves administering a series of shock waves directly to a painful tendon. Its proposed mechanism of action is disruption of neoneuralization found in tendinopathic tissue that may be linked to symptomatic pain.[42] There has also been evidence linking ESWT administration to increased tenocyte proliferation, which would benefit the healing process of an injured tendon.[43]

As with many other forms of treatment for tendinopathy, supporting evidence is either limited or contradictory. A review of recent placebo-controlled trials focusing on various forms of tendinopathy included 3 studies. Each reported significant differences in favor of ESWT in nearly all outcome measures examined.[44-46] Five separate studies, however, reported no benefit in the use of ESWT.[47-51]

A randomized, controlled trial from Rompe and coworkers[41] compared ESWT with eccentric strengthening exercises in 50 patients with insertional Achilles tendinopathy.[41] By 4 months, the group receiving ESWT reported 64% improvement compared

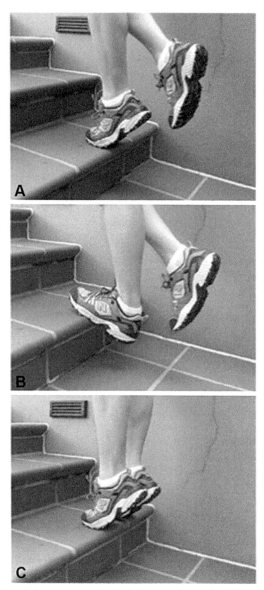

Fig. 3. An eccentric training program for Achilles tendinopathy. (*A*) The patient starts in a single-leg standing position with the weight on the forefoot and the ankle in full plantar flexion. (*B*) The Achilles is then eccentrically loaded by slowly lowering the heel to a dorsiflexed position. (*C*) The patient then returns to the starting position using the arms or contralateral leg for assistance to avoid concentric loading of the involved Achilles tendon. (*From* Andres BM, Murrell GA. Treatment of tendinopathy: what works, what doesn't and what's on the horizon. Clin Orthop Relat Res 2008;466:1541; with permission.)

with 28% in the eccentric exercise group with regard to pain, general outcomes, and Achilles-specific scores. Another recent randomized, controlled trial performed by Cacchio and colleagues[52] examined ESWT compared with conservative management with NSAIDs and physical therapy in 40 cases of proximal hamstring tendinopathy. After 3 months of treatment, 85% of patients receiving ESWT had at least a 50% reduction in pain symptoms compared with only 10% of patients in the conservative group.

Nonetheless, there continues to be considerable debate regarding the use of ESWT in the treatment of tendinopathy. Controversy exists in almost all aspects of its use, from dosing regimens to patient-directed targeting of therapy to the site of maximal tenderness versus imaged-guided therapy with fluoroscopy or ultrasound.[52] Even concurrent use of local anesthesia seems to have an effect on outcomes, with one study paradoxically showing significantly lower success rates from therapy that used a local anesthetic during administration of ESWT.[53] Given the overall discordance in evidence, the use of ESWT in treatment of tendinopathy cannot be definitively recommended as a first-line treatment and should be reserved only for patients recalcitrant to other conservative methods such as eccentric exercises or corticosteroid injections.[47,54]

INJECTION THERAPY

Injectable substances have been used in the treatment of tendinopathy for decades, first reaching widespread acceptance with the use of corticosteroids when it was believed, albeit incorrectly, that an inflammatory process was the underlying cause of symptoms. This avenue of therapy has since evolved to include myriad options, including autologous whole blood injections, platelet-rich plasma, and injectable sclerosing agents. Promising results have been shown; however, investigations are of varied design and quality. Difficulty still remains to definitively recommend injections as first-line treatment.

Autologous Whole Blood

The use of autologous whole blood as an injectable agent in the treatment of tendinopathy is a relatively new avenue of therapy. Its focus is on augmenting the in vivo biological processes that are at play during the body's response to tendon degeneration and wear, leading to quicker recovery and more robust healing.[55–57]

Injection of autologous whole blood aims to promote tendon healing by stimulating a well-organized angiogenic response and subsequent collagen regeneration.[58] The key to its therapeutic potential stems from the host of growth factors and proteins found in its milieu. Two of these factors, transforming growth factor-β (TGF-β) and fibroblast growth factor, have been shown to act as humeral mediators, inducing the healing cascade in injured tendons.[55,59]

Five studies recently investigated the use of autologous whole blood as an injection therapy: 1 involving patellar tendinopathy and 4 focusing on elbow epicondylosis. Kazemi and colleagues[60] performed a randomized, controlled trial of 60 cases of lateral epicondylosis divided equally into treatment groups receiving either an injection of autologous whole blood or a corticosteroid. At the end of an 8-week follow up period, all outcomes, including pain score and grip strength, were significantly improved in those receiving whole blood injections. These promising results come in the setting of some limitations, however, including a relatively short follow-up period as well as blinding of only the assessors and not the treatment group patients themselves.

The remaining 4 studies investigating the benefit of autologous whole blood injection as a treatment for tendinopathy were all prospective case series.[56,61–63] Even though all studies did report improvement in pain and function after injection, these results are difficult to interpret in the setting of a case series, as the results cannot be definitively attributed to the injection because there is no control group to offer comparison. As such, there is limited overall evidence to assess the efficacy of autologous whole blood injection in the treatment of tendinopathy.

Platelet-Rich Plasma

Platelet-rich plasma (PRP) offers another avenue of therapy that intends to augment the native healing at the site of tendon injury through the exogenous addition of biological factors. Since the 1980s, PRP has been the focus of study with regard to its purported benefit to soft tissue healing and bone regeneration.[64] Throughout that time, its investigational applications have expanded to include chronic muscle strains, fibrosis, ligamentous sprains, rotator cuff injuries, joint capsular laxity, and tendinopathy.[65–72]

PRP is prepared from autologous whole blood, which is then centrifuged to concentrate the platelets in a plasma background.[58,73] Laboratory studies have found platelets to contain a high concentration of growth factors including TGF-β, fibroblast growth factor-2, platelet-derived growth factor, insulin-like growth factor, vascular endothelial growth factor, epidermal growth factor, and connective tissue growth factor.[64] These factors have been found to play vital roles in stimulating mesenchymal cell proliferation, collagen synthesis, and angiogenesis—all important processes in the maintenance and repair of tendon tissue.[73–76] The rationale for the use of PRP in treatment of tendinopathy, therefore, is the ability to deliver hyerphysiologic doses of beneficial growth factors directly to the site of tendon pathology.

There has been substantially more research dedicated to PRP in the treatment of tendinopathy than autologous whole blood. Two recent double-blind, randomized, controlled trials investigated the effects of PRP injections on Achilles tendinopathy and lateral epicondylitis, respectively. De Vos and colleagues[77] looked at 54 cases of Achilles tendinopathy and compared the effect of PRP injection with that of a placebo injection. Both treatment groups also underwent a concurrent eccentric exercise program. At 6-month follow-up, both groups exhibited significant improvements in patient satisfaction and return to sport. There was no difference in outcome measures, however, when comparing the 2 treatment groups directly. Peerbooms and coworkers[78] performed a second randomized controlled trial in which PRP injection was compared with corticosteroid injection in 100 cases of lateral epicondylitis and found contrasting results. At 12-month follow-up, outcome measures were significantly improved in the PRP group with an overall success rate of 73% compared with 49% in the steroid group.

Additional high-quality randomized, controlled trials investigating PRP injections for tendinopathy are lacking. Two recent nonrandomized trials, however, also showed contrasting results in terms of the efficacy of PRP injections.[65,79] Filardo and coworkers[79] examined 31 cases of patellar tendinopathy treated with either PRP injection and physical therapy or physical therapy alone. Their group found improvements in overall outcome measures, but there was no significant difference detected when comparing the 2 treatment groups. These 2 studies would appear to lend more credence to the benefit of physical therapy rather than the use of PRP.

Mishra and Pavelko[65] performed a second nonrandomized clinical trial looking at 20 cases of lateral epicondylitis and compared the use of PRP with injections of bupivacaine with epinephrine. At 8 weeks there was a significant improvement in pain and function in the PRP group compared with the bupivacaine group. Unfortunately, the small cohort of 20 patients with short-term follow-up may hamper the impact of this study.

In addition to the studies mentioned above, there has been a host of prospective case studies aimed at determining the benefit of PRP injections on various forms of tendinopathy, including patellar and Achilles. The majority of these show improvements in pain, function, and patient satisfaction after injection.[68,80] Again, this evidence must be looked at objectively, however, because of the inherent design limitations of prospective case studies lacking control groups for comparison.

The use of PRP as an injection therapy for treatment of tendinopathy shows great promise. Further study with additional high-quality randomized, controlled trials is necessary before the efficacy can be determined definitively. At press time, the American Academy of Orthopaedic Surgeons has commissioned the 2011 PRP Study Group[81] (http://www.aaos.org/news/acadnews/2011/AAOS1_2_16.asp). Fifty national and international orthopaedic and musculoskeletal experts are charged with determining the efficacy of PRP and developing manufacturing standards for industry. The committee results are highly anticipated and expected to guide indications for future PRP utilization.

Corticosteroids

Corticosteroids have long been a mainstay in the treatment of tendinopathy, initially chosen for their anti-inflammatory effects. Despite current knowledge that inflammation plays much less of a role in tendinopathy than originally thought, steroids have maintained their status as a first-line intervention. One hypothesis for their proposed efficacy is that the degenerative change seen within affected tendons causes an inflammatory response in the surrounding tissue that may contribute to pain and swelling seen in cases of tendinopathy.[82] In this setting, steroids would serve to offer symptomatic relief but not necessarily address the underlying pathologic cause. Recent literature seems to corroborate this notion, often showing short-term improvements in symptoms with few long-term benefits.

A classically cited randomized, controlled trial evaluated the effects of steroid injections, eccentric exercises, and resistance training in the setting of patellar tendinopathy. Within the first 6 months of follow-up, all 3 treatment arms showed significant improvement in patient outcomes (pain and functional improvement).[83] After that period; however, the eccentric and resistance training groups were shown to maintain their positive benefits while symptomatic relief deteriorated in the steroid injection group.

Other randomized, controlled trials, one comparing steroid with aprotinin (a proteinase inhibitor) injection in cases of patellar tendinopathy and another comparing steroid injection with observation or physical therapy in cases of lateral epicondylitis, have shown similar results: initial improvement in outcomes in the steroid group but with tapering long-term benefits.[84]

Indeed, the majority of evidence available calls into question the long-term efficacy of corticosteroid injections for the treatment of tendinopathy.[20,85-89] Aside from this question in efficacy, safety concerns have also been raised. Several cases of Achilles tendon rupture have been reported after corticosteroid injection.[89-92] According to Gill and colleagues,[93] safe and efficacious peritendinous Achilles injections are possible with fluoroscopic assistance to ensure delivery around the tendon rather than within its substance.

Overall, the injection of corticosteroid as a treatment for tendinopathy appears to offer consistent short-term pain relief, but there is little evidence as to longer-term benefit.

Sclerosing Agents

Research into the pathophysiology of tendinopathy has shown an increase in neoneurovascularization in affected tendon tissue.[94,95] It is believed that this increase in neural density contributes to the pain felt during active disease.[96-98] This hypothesis forms the basis for sclerotherapy, where injectable caustic agents aim to destroy neovessels and their accompanying nervous structures, reducing overall pain symptoms.

Polidocanol, an injectable sclerosing agent, has long been used to treat varicose veins and telangiectasias.[99] It has also become the main agent used in studies investigating the effect of sclerosing agents in cases of tendinopathy, including several reports in case series and multiple randomized, controlled trials.

Three separate double-blinded randomized, controlled trials have been performed comparing polidocanol injection with a placebo injection containing lidocaine and adrenaline in the setting of lateral epicondylitis (n = 34), patellar tendinopathy (n = 42), and Achilles tendinopathy (n = 20), respectively.[100-102] Follow-up ranged from between 3 and 12 months. The studies investigating patellar and Achilles tendinopathy showed significant improvement in patient outcomes (pain with tendon loading and patient satisfaction) in the sclerosing group compared with placebo. In contrast, however, the lateral epicondylitis trial did not show any differences between the 2 treatment groups.

Eight different prospective case trials were examined for this review, running the gamut of lateral epicondylar, patellar, Achilles, extensor pollicis brevis, and abductor pollicis tendinopathy. All showed promising results in the form of improved patient outcome scores after polidocanol injection.[101,103-111] It is important to once again point out the limitations of such studies, however, in that there is no placebo group to offer comparison within each trial. Following suit with other research on injection therapies for tendinopathy, the use of sclerosing agents seems to offer great promise but currently lacks enough high-quality evidence to garner definitive recommendation.

Aprotinin

Matrix metalloproteinases (MMPs) are a large family of enzymes that work to degrade tendon matrix components and play a vital role during development and tendon repair.[112,113] Recent basic science research has shown an increase in MMPs in tendinopathic tissue and, as such, these enzymes may be key effectors of the pathologic processes in chronic tendon disease, causing delayed tendon healing and clinical recovery.[114,115]

Early research has begun to look at the injection of aprotinin, a proteinase inhibitor, as a possible therapeutic intervention to counteract the excessive MMP action in the setting of tendinopathy. In a retrospective cohort study, Orchard and colleagues[116] determined that in major load-bearing tendons (ie, Achilles, patella, hamstring), aprotinin is not as effective as corticosteroid injection and therefore should be thought of as a second-line injection option.[84,116] Although the involvement of MMPs in tendinopathy seems to offer an interesting avenue of study from a basic science standpoint, the clinical use of aprotinin clearly requires further study before any meaningful conclusions can be drawn.

Prolotherapy

Prolotherapy, or the use of high-volume injection as a treatment for tendinopathy, is a resurgent modality receiving renewed interest. Originally described by a general surgeon in the 1950s, proliferants are injected at the site of injury or pain and are purported to induce an inflammatory response.[117] Three commonly used solutions act via distinctly different mechanisms. Dextrose causes osmotic cellular rupture, phenol-glycerine-glucose by local cellular irritation, and sodium morrhuate by chemotactic attraction of inflammatory mediators.[118]

Early reports attempted to validate prolotherapy as a panacea for all musculoskeletal ailments. A systematic review of 42 prolotherapy studies (including osteoarthritis, low back pain, and overuse conditions) was unable to determine which patients would benefit most from prolotherapy.[119] Another report found clinical success with prolotherapy for lateral epicondylitis, although the study may have been limited by small patient groups.[117] A recent meta-analysis reviewed the efficacy of injection therapy for tendinopathy, including 2 studies on prolotherapy.[120] Prolotherapy was shown to reduce pain associated with lateral epicondylitis in the intermediate term and was also more effective than eccentric exercises in relieving pain associated with Achilles tendinopathy. Certainly, further study is warranted to validate the use of alternative injection therapy before widespread clinical adoption of the techniques.

OPERATIVE MANAGEMENT

The use of operative management for treatment of tendinopathy focuses on the excision of fibrotic adhesions and areas of affected tendon that have failed to heal. Ultimately, the aim is to restore vascularity and stimulate viable tenocytes to initiate protein synthesis and promote repair.[121,122] A recent study has found that tenotomies made in Achilles tendon did indeed trigger angiogenesis and increased blood flow, lending credence to the idea that surgical intervention can help create a more favorable environment for healing.[123]

Multiple operative methods for the management of tendinopathy have been reported. Open debridement is the most commonly reported method, and, once again, results vary widely from study to study. In a retrospective study performed by Morberg and colleagues, only 67% of patients treated with open debridement for Achilles tendinopathy reported improvement in symptoms and return to function at a mean follow-up of 6 years.[124] Several other studies have reported similar subjective improvement in those with Achilles tendinopathy. Significantly improved outcomes, however; have only been found in patients who had chronic peritendinopathy.[8,125] This would seem to indicate that the extent of tendon pathology and involvement has some bearing on the efficacy of surgical intervention.

A recent observational study investigated the arthroscopic management of chronic patellar tendinopathy. Twenty-three patients with tendinopathy that was unresponsive to conservative management underwent arthroscopic debridement with a minimum of 12 months of follow-up. A significant improvement in patient outcomes was seen matching previously published data on open debridement of the patella tendon.[126] A similar conclusion was established in several case series by Baker[127] and Grewal and coworkers[128] looking at arthroscopic management of lateral epicondylitis.

Lattermann and colleagues[129] recently reported on 36 patients treated with arthroscopic debridement of the extensor carpi radialis brevis origin for recalcitrant lateral epicondylitis. All patients had failed nonoperative treatment and underwent surgery, on average, 19 months after symptom onset. At 3-year follow-up the Mayo Clinic elbow score was 11.1, and pain had improved in 96%.

In further efforts to define suitable minimally invasive techniques for operative management, percutaneous longitudinal tenotomies have been reported to be effective in cases of isolated tendinopathy with a well-defined lesion under 2.5 cm in length.[130] This can be performed in the ambulatory setting under local anesthesia and with the aid of ultrasound guidance for precise localization of pathology.[130,131] Endoscopic-assisted surgical treatment has also been described. Tendoscopy has been described for use in the ankle to gain access to posterior tibial, peroneal, and

Achilles tendons.[132–134] There are limited data supporting this technique, but a study by Thermann and coworkers[135] reported good short-term clinical results in 8 cases of Achilles tendinopathy.

Although there is evidence supporting surgical intervention for cases of chronic tendinopathy, predicting which patients will have continued problems postoperatively is difficult. Treatment failure rates can be as high as 20% to 30%.[136] For this reason, surgical intervention should be held as a last resort for only those patients who have not responded to an extensive course of conservative management.

AUTHORS' PREFERRED TECHNIQUE

Achilles tendinopathy is a common cause of pain and disability in the running athlete and ranks among the most common conditions found in athletic training rooms and sports medicine clinics. While the mainstay of treatment is conservative, each treatment regimen ought to be customized to the athlete and his/her sport.

Initial treatment is centered on pain control and reducing inflammation. Relative rest from running, ice, elevation and compression are helpful acutely. We discourage our running athletes from hill and interval workouts for 3–5 days. Aerobic conditioning is maintained with swimming and/or stationary cycling so long as athletes remain asymptomatic. A five-day course of anti-inflammatory medication (naproxen sodium 500mg twice daily) is often helpful. Collegiate running athletes are instructed in a gastrocnemius-soleus stretching program including ankle range of motion and eccentric exercises as described above. Achilles strengthening is begun once symptoms have improved and continued throughout the season.

Transdermal glycerol trinitrate patches (Nitro-Dur, Merck & Co., Inc. Whitehouse Station, NJ, USA) are prescribed for athletes with recurrent pain. One-quarter patch is applied daily to the point of maximal tenderness. Advanced imaging with MRI is reserved for athletes who fail early conservative treatment.

We do not routinely use corticosteroid injections in our athletes with Achilles tendinosis. Alternatively, we have found success with platelet-rich plasma injections.

Fluoroscopically guided injections are performed with radio-opaque dye (Visipaque, GE Healthcare, Little Chalfont, United Kingdom) diluted 1:4 with sterile saline. The tendon is localized with a dye injection and platelet-rich plasma concentrate is injected (**Fig. 4**). Patients are restricted from running for 7 days and instructed with ankle range of motion exercises.

Operative treatment is reserved only for the most recalcitrant cases in athletes who have failed 3–6 months of conservative treatment. A paramedian incision is made with the patient positioned prone. The tendon sheath is opened longitudinally and adhesions to the peritenon are released. Nodular, degenerative regions within the tendon are debrided and excised through a longitudinal split in the mid-substance. A side-to-side tendon repair is performed in most patients. When debridement and excision exceed 25% of the tendon an end-to-end repair may be necessary. Post-operatively patients are immobilized in a removable walking boot for 2 weeks. Daily ankle range of motion exercises are begun immediately and regimented Achilles rehabilitation commences once immobilization is discontinued.

SUMMARY

Tendinopathy is a common and debilitating condition that results in significant deficits in performance and prolonged time away from activity. For this reason, much effort has been placed in defining beneficial and cost-effective treatments. This review has outlined the current literature on some of the most widely used therapies for cases of tendinopathy. As such, recommendations remain limited by the evidence available.

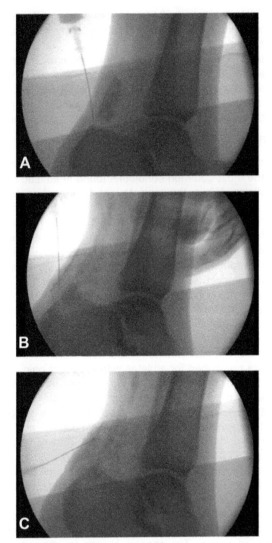

Fig. 4. PRP injection under fluoroscopy. (*A*) Localization of the retrocalcaneal bursa with injection of radio-opaque dye. The needle is repositioned within the tendon at the insertion (*B*) and in the proximal mid-substance (*C*).

The variability in both quantity and quality of research into tendinopathy treatments makes it difficult to make definitive treatment recommendations. In general, however, a reasonable first line of treatment for tendinopathy should include a course of NSAIDs and eccentric exercise-based physical therapy. Corticosteroid injections seem to offer excellent short-term pain relief but lack long term efficacy. Alternative injections, such as PRP, have shown short-term efficacy for tendinopathy sufferers; data are lacking to support sclerosing agents and proteinase inhibitors. Operative management seems to offer some benefit in symptomatic relief but carries a higher complication rate than other treatment options and should be reserved only for patients recalcitrant to other more conservative options.

Although the inability to make definitive therapeutic recommendations in some instances is discouraging, it is important to note that a lack of high-quality evidence supporting specific treatments does not necessarily imply that they are inherently ineffective. Given the growing prevalence of tendinopathy and the impact it has on the general public, it is more important now than ever to continue the search for the most effective and accessible treatment modalities.

REFERENCES

1. Hreljac A, Marshall RN, Hume PA. Evaluation of lower extremity overuse injury potential in runners. Med Sci Sports Exerc 2000;32(9):1635–41.
2. Hreljac A. Impact and overuse injuries in runners. Med Sci Sports Exerc 2004;36(5): 845–9.
3. Taunton JE, Ryan MB, Clement DB, et al. A retrospective case-control analysis of 2002 running injuries. Br J Sports Med 2002;36(2):95–101.
4. Abate M, Silbernagel KG, Siljeholm C, et al. Pathogenesis of tendinopathies: inflammation or degeneration? Arthritis Res Ther 2009;11(3):235.
5. Fu SC, Rolf C, Cheuk YC, et al. Deciphering the pathogenesis of tendinopathy: a three-stages process. Sports Med Arthrosc Rehabil Ther Technol 2010;2:30.
6. Longo UG, Rittweger J, Garau G, et al. No influence of age, gender, weight, height, and impact profile in achilles tendinopathy in masters track and field athletes. Am J Sports Med 2009;37(7):1400–5.
7. Khan KM, Scott A. Mechanotherapy: how physical therapists' prescription of exercise promotes tissue repair. Br J Sports Med. 2009;43(4):247–52.
8. Lian OB, Engebretsen L, Bahr R. Prevalence of jumper's knee among elite athletes from different sports: a cross-sectional study. Am J Sports Med 2005;33(4):561–7.
9. Gardin A, Movin T, Svensson L, et al. The long-term clinical and MRI results following eccentric calf muscle training in chronic Achilles tendinosis. Skeletal Radiol 2010; 39(5):435–42.
10. Magnussen RA, Dunn WR, Thomson AB. Nonoperative treatment of midportion Achilles tendinopathy: a systematic review. Clin J Sport Med 2009;19(1):54–64.
11. Paavola M, Kannus P, Paakkala T, et al. Long-term prognosis of patients with achilles tendinopathy. An observational 8-year follow-up study. Am J Sports Med 2000;28(5):634–42.
12. Magra M, Maffulli N. Nonsteroidal antiinflammatory drugs in tendinopathy: friend or foe. Clin J Sport Med 2006;16(1):1–3.
13. Magra M, Maffulli N. Genetic aspects of tendinopathy. J Sci Med Sport 2008;11(3): 243–7.
14. Aström M, Westlin N. No effect of piroxicam on achilles tendinopathy. A randomized study of 70 patients. Acta orthopaedica Scandinavica 1992;63(6):631–4.
15. Spacca G, Cacchio A, Forgacs A, et al. Analgesic efficacy of a lecithin-vehiculated diclofenac epolamine gel in shoulder periarthritis and lateral epicondylitis: a placebo-controlled, multicenter, randomized, double-blind clinical trial. Drugs Exp Clin Res 2005;31(4):147–54.
16. Petri M, Hufman SL, Waser G, et al. Celecoxib effectively treats patients with acute shoulder tendinitis/bursitis. J Rheumatol 2004;31(8):1614–20.
17. Mazieres B, Rouanet S, Guillon Y, et al. Topical ketoprofen patch in the treatment of tendinitis: a randomized, double blind, placebo controlled study. J Rheumatol 2005;32(8):1563–70.
18. Lopez JM. Treatment of acute tendinitis and bursitis with fentiazac—a double-blind comparison with placebo. Clin Ther 1982;5(1):79–84.

19. Labelle H, Guibert R. Efficacy of diclofenac in lateral epicondylitis of the elbow also treated with immobilization. The University of Montreal Orthopaedic Research Group. Arch Fam Med 1997;6(3):257–62.
20. Hay EM, Paterson SM, Lewis M, et al. Pragmatic randomised controlled trial of local corticosteroid injection and naproxen for treatment of lateral epicondylitis of elbow in primary care. BMJ 1999;319(7215):964–8.
21. Paoloni JA, Appleyard RC, Nelson J, et al. Topical nitric oxide application in the treatment of chronic extensor tendinosis at the elbow: a randomized, double-blinded, placebo-controlled clinical trial. Am J Sports Med 2003;31(6):915–20.
22. Murrell GA. Oxygen free radicals and tendon healing. J Shoulder Elbow Surg 2007;16(5 Suppl):S208–14.
23. Murrell GA, Szabo C, Hannafin JA, et al. Modulation of tendon healing by nitric oxide. Inflamm Res 1997;46(1):19–27.
24. Paoloni JA, Appleyard RC, Nelson J, et al. Topical glyceryl trinitrate application in the treatment of chronic supraspinatus tendinopathy: a randomized, double-blinded, placebo-controlled clinical trial. Am J Sports Med 2005;33(6):806–13.
25. Paoloni JA, Murrell GA, Burch RM, et al. Randomised, double-blind, placebo-controlled clinical trial of a new topical glyceryl trinitrate patch for chronic lateral epicondylosis. Br J Sports Med 2009;43(4):299–302.
26. Pons S, Gallardo C, Caballero J, et al. [Transdermal nitroglycerin versus corticosteroid infiltration for rotator cuff tendinitis]. Aten Primaria 2001;28(7):452–5[in Spanish].
27. Berrazueta JR, Losada A, Poveda J, et al. Successful treatment of shoulder pain syndrome due to supraspinatus tendinitis with transdermal nitroglycerin. A double blind study. Pain 1996;66(1):63–7.
28. Kane TP, Ismail M, Calder JD. Topical glyceryl trinitrate and noninsertional Achilles tendinopathy: a clinical and cellular investigation. Am J Sports Med 2008;36(6):1160–3.
29. Gambito ED, Gonzalez-Suarez CB, Oquinena TI, et al. Evidence of the effectiveness of topical nitroglycerin in the treatment of tendinopathies: a systematic review and meta-analysis. Arch Phys Med Rehabili 2010;91(8):1291–305.
30. McCallum SD, Paoloni JA, Murrell GA. Five-year prospective comparison study of topical glyceryl trinitrate treatment of chronic lateral epicondylosis at the elbow. Br J Sports Med 2011;45(5):416–20.
31. Lorenz D, Reiman M. The role and implementation of eccentric training in athletic rehabilitation: tendinopathy, hamstring strains, and acl reconstruction. Int J Sports Phys Ther 2011;6(1):27–44.
32. Shalabi A, Kristoffersen-Wilberg M, Svensson L, et al. Eccentric training of the gastrocnemius-soleus complex in chronic Achilles tendinopathy results in decreased tendon volume and intratendinous signal as evaluated by MRI. Am J Sports Med 2004;32(5):1286–96.
33. Langberg H, Ellingsgaard H, Madsen T, et al. Eccentric rehabilitation exercise increases peritendinous type I collagen synthesis in humans with Achilles tendinosis. Scand J Med Sci Sports 2007;17(1):61–6.
34. Norregaard J, Larsen CC, Bieler T, et al. Eccentric exercise in treatment of Achilles tendinopathy. Scand J Med Sci Sports 2007;17(2):133–8.
35. Rompe JD, Nafe B, Furia JP, et al. Eccentric loading, shock-wave treatment, or a wait-and-see policy for tendinopathy of the main body of tendo Achillis: a randomized controlled trial. Am J Sports Med 2007;35(3):374–83.
36. Jonsson P, Alfredson H. Superior results with eccentric compared to concentric quadriceps training in patients with jumper's knee: a prospective randomised study. Br J Sports Med 2005;39(11):847–50.

37. Young MA, Cook JL, Purdam CR, et al. Eccentric decline squat protocol offers superior results at 12 months compared with traditional eccentric protocol for patellar tendinopathy in volleyball players. Br J Sports Med 2005;39(2):102–5.
38. Roos EM, Engstrom M, Lagerquist A, et al. Clinical improvement after 6 weeks of eccentric exercise in patients with mid-portion Achilles tendinopathy—a randomized trial with 1-year follow-up. Scand J Med Sci Sports 2004;14(5):286–95.
39. Mafi N, Lorentzon R, Alfredson H. Superior short-term results with eccentric calf muscle training compared to concentric training in a randomized prospective multicenter study on patients with chronic Achilles tendinosis. Knee Surg Sports Traumatol Arthrosc 2001;9(1):42–7.
40. Silbernagel KG, Brorsson A, Lundberg M. The majority of patients with Achilles tendinopathy recover fully when treated with exercise alone: a 5-year follow-up. Am J Sports Med 2011;39(3):607–13.
41. Rompe JD, Furia J, Maffulli N. Eccentric loading compared with shock wave treatment for chronic insertional achilles tendinopathy. A randomized, controlled trial. J Bone Joint Surg 2008;90(1):52–61.
42. Crisp T, Khan F, Padhiar N, et al. High volume ultrasound guided injections at the interface between the patellar tendon and Hoffa's body are effective in chronic patellar tendinopathy: a pilot study. Disabil Rehabil 2008;30(20–22):1625–34.
43. Ohtori S, Inoue G, Mannoji C, et al. Shock wave application to rat skin induces degeneration and reinnervation of sensory nerve fibres. Neurosci Lett 2001; 315(1-2):57–60.
44. Chen YJ, Wang CJ, Yang KD, et al. Extracorporeal shock waves promote healing of collagenase-induced Achilles tendinitis and increase TGF-beta1 and IGF-I expression. J Orthop Res 2004;22(4):854–61.
45. Rompe JD, Hope C, Kullmer K, et al. Analgesic effect of extracorporeal shock-wave therapy on chronic tennis elbow. J Bone Joint Surg Br 1996;78(2):233–7.
46. Rompe JD, Decking J, Schoellner C, et al. Repetitive low-energy shock wave treatment for chronic lateral epicondylitis in tennis players. Am J Sports Med 2004;32(3):734–43.
47. Pettrone FA, McCall BR. Extracorporeal shock wave therapy without local anesthesia for chronic lateral epicondylitis. J Bone Joint Surg Am 2005;87(6):1297–304.
48. Haake M, Konig IR, Decker T, et al. Extracorporeal shock wave therapy in the treatment of lateral epicondylitis: a randomized multicenter trial. J Bone Joint Surg Am 2002;84–A(11):1982–91.
49. Speed CA, Nichols D, Richards C, et al. Extracorporeal shock wave therapy for lateral epicondylitis—a double blind randomised controlled trial. J Orthop Res 2002;20(5):895–8.
50. Melikyan EY, Shahin E, Miles J, et al. Extracorporeal shock-wave treatment for tennis elbow. A randomised double-blind study. J Bone Joint Surg Br 2003;85(6):852–5.
51. Chung B, Wiley JP. Effectiveness of extracorporeal shock wave therapy in the treatment of previously untreated lateral epicondylitis: a randomized controlled trial. Am J Sports Med 2004;32(7):1660–7.
52. Cacchio A, Rompe JD, Furia JP, et al. Shockwave therapy for the treatment of chronic proximal hamstring tendinopathy in professional athletes. Am J Sports Med 2011;39(1):146–53.
53. Buchbinder R, Green Shock wave therapy for lateral elbow pain. Cochrane Database Syst Rev 2005;4:CD003524.
54. Labek G, Auersperg V, Ziernhold M, et al. [Influence of local anesthesia and energy level on the clinical outcome of extracorporeal shock wave-treatment of chronic plantar fasciitis]. Z Orthop Ihre Grenzgeb 2005;143(2):240–6[in German].

55. Iwasaki M, Nakahara H, Nakata K, et al. Regulation of proliferation and osteochondrogenic differentiation of periosteum-derived cells by transforming growth factor-beta and basic fibroblast growth factor. J Bone Joint Surg Am 1995;77(4):543–54.

56. Edwards SG, Calandruccio JH. Autologous blood injections for refractory lateral epicondylitis. J Hand Surg Am 2003;28(2):272–8.

57. Taylor MA, Norman TL, Clovis NB, et al. The response of rabbit patellar tendons after autologous blood injection. Med Sci Sports Exerc 2002;34(1):70–3.

58. de Vos RJ, van Veldhoven PL, Moen MH, et al. Autologous growth factor injections in chronic tendinopathy: a systematic review. Br Med Bull 2010;95:63–77.

59. Rabago D, Best TM, Zgierska AE, et al. A systematic review of four injection therapies for lateral epicondylosis: prolotherapy, polidocanol, whole blood and platelet-rich plasma. Br J Sports Med 2009;43(7):471–81.

60. Kazemi M, Azma K, Tavana B, Rezaiee Moghaddam F, et al. Autologous blood versus corticosteroid local injection in the short-term treatment of lateral elbow tendinopathy: a randomized clinical trial of efficacy. Am J Phys Med Rehabil 2010; 89(8):660–7.

61. Connell DA, Ali KE, Ahmad M, et al. Ultrasound-guided autologous blood injection for tennis elbow. Skeletal Radiol 2006;35(6):371–7.

62. James SL, Ali K, Pocock C, et al. Ultrasound guided dry needling and autologous blood injection for patellar tendinosis. Br J Sports Med 2007;41(8):518–21[discussion: 522].

63. Suresh SP, Ali KE, Jones H, et al. Medial epicondylitis: is ultrasound guided autologous blood injection an effective treatment? Br J Sports Med 2006;40(11): 935–9[discussion: 939].

64. Everts PA, Knape JT, Weibrich G, et al. Platelet-rich plasma and platelet gel: a review. J Extra Corpor Technol 2006;38(2):174–87.

65. Mishra A, Pavelko T. Treatment of chronic elbow tendinosis with buffered platelet-rich plasma. Am J Sports Med 2006;34(11):1774–8.

66. Gamradt SC, Rodeo SA, Warren RF. Platelet rich plasma in rotator cuff repair. Techniques in Orthopaedics 2007;22(1):26–33.

67. Randelli PS, Arrigoni P, Cabitza P, et al. Autologous platelet rich plasma for arthroscopic rotator cuff repair. A pilot study. Disabil Rehabil 2008;30(20–22):1584–9.

68. Kon E, Filardo G, Delcogliano M, et al. Platelet-rich plasma: new clinical application: a pilot study for treatment of jumper's knee. Injury 2009;40(6):598–603.

69. Foster TE, Puskas BL, Mandelbaum BR, et al. Platelet-rich plasma: from basic science to clinical applications. Am J Sports Med 2009;37(11):2259–72.

70. Sanchez M, Anitua E, Orive G, et al. Platelet-rich therapies in the treatment of orthopaedic sport injuries. Sports Med 2009;39(5):345–54.

71. Sampson S, Gerhardt M, Mandelbaum B. Platelet rich plasma injection grafts for musculoskeletal injuries: a review. Curr Rev Musculoskelet Med 2008;1(3-4): 165–74.

72. Hall MP, Band PA, Meislin RJ, et al. Platelet-rich plasma: current concepts and application in sports medicine. J Am Acad Orthop Surg 2009;17(10):602–8.

73. Mishra A, Woodall J Jr, Vieira A. Treatment of tendon and muscle using platelet-rich plasma. Clin Sports Med 2009;28(1):113–25.

74. Sharma P, Maffulli N. Biology of tendon injury: healing, modeling and remodeling. J Musculoskelet Neuronal Interact 2006;6(2):181–90.

75. Sharma P, Maffulli N. Basic biology of tendon injury and healing. Surgeon 2005;3(5): 309–16.

76. Sharma P, Maffulli N. Tendinopathy and tendon injury: the future. Disabil Rehabil 2008;30(20–22):1733–45.

77. de Vos RJ, Weir A, van Schie HT, et al. Platelet-rich plasma injection for chronic Achilles tendinopathy: a randomized controlled trial. JAMA 2010;303(2):144–9.

78. Peerbooms JC, Sluimer J, Bruijn DJ, et al. Positive effect of an autologous platelet concentrate in lateral epicondylitis in a double-blind randomized controlled trial: platelet-rich plasma versus corticosteroid injection with a 1-year follow-up. Am J Sports Med 2010;38(2):255–62.

79. Filardo G, Kon E, Della Villa S, et al. Use of platelet-rich plasma for the treatment of refractory jumper's knee. Int Orthop 2010;34(6):909–15.

80. Fredberg U, Bolvig L, Pfeiffer-Jensen M, et al. Ultrasonography as a tool for diagnosis, guidance of local steroid injection and, together with pressure algometry, monitoring of the treatment of athletes with chronic jumper's knee and Achilles tendinitis: a randomized, double-blind, placebo-controlled study. Scand J Rheumatol 2004;33(2):94–101.

81. PRP: An unproven option, say experts. 2011. Available at: www.aaos.org/news/acadnews/2011/AAOS1_2_16.asp. Accessed October 23, 2011.

82. Kongsgaard M, Kovanen V, Aagaard P, et al. Corticosteroid injections, eccentric decline squat training and heavy slow resistance training in patellar tendinopathy. Scand J Med Sci Sports 2009;19(6):790–802.

83. Capasso G, Testa V, Maffulli N. Aprotinin, corticosteroids and normosaline in the management of patellar tendinopathy in athletes: a prospective randomized study. Injury 1997;3(2):111–5.

84. Tonks JH, Pai SK, Murali SR. Steroid injection therapy is the best conservative treatment for lateral epicondylitis: a prospective randomised controlled trial. Int J Clin Pract 2007;61(2):240–6.

85. Smidt N, Assendelft WJ, van der Windt DA, et al. Corticosteroid injections for lateral epicondylitis: a systematic review. Pain 2002;96(1-2):23–40.

86. Smidt N, van der Windt DA, Assendelft WJ, et al. Corticosteroid injections, physiotherapy, or a wait-and-see policy for lateral epicondylitis: a randomised controlled trial. Lancet 23 2002;359(9307):657–62.

87. Verhaar JA, Walenkamp GH, van Mameren H, et al. Local corticosteroid injection versus Cyriax-type physiotherapy for tennis elbow. J Bone Joint Surg Br 1996;78(1):128–32.

88. Barr S, Cerisola FL, Blanchard V. Effectiveness of corticosteroid injections compared with physiotherapeutic interventions for lateral epicondylitis: a systematic review. Physiotherapy 2009;95(4):251–65.

89. Kleinman M, Gross AE. Achilles tendon rupture following steroid injection. Report of three cases. J Bone Joint Surg Am 1983;65(9):1345–7.

90. Ford LT, DeBender J. Tendon rupture after local steroid injection. South Med J 1979;72(7):827–30.

91. Jones JG. Achilles tendon rupture following steroid injection. J Bone Joint Surg Am 1985;67(1):170.

92. Chechick A, Amit Y, Israeli A, et al. Recurrent rupture of the achilles tendon induced by corticosteroid injection. Br J Sports Med 1982;16(2):89–90.

93. Gill SS, Gelbke MK, Mattson SL, et al. Fluoroscopically guided low-volume peritendinous corticosteroid injection for Achilles tendinopathy. A safety study. J Bone Joint Surg Am 2004;86-A(4):802–6.

94. Ohberg L, Lorentzon R, Alfredson H. Neovascularisation in Achilles tendons with painful tendinosis but not in normal tendons: an ultrasonographic investigation. Knee Surg Sports Traumatol Arthrosc 2001;9(4):233–8.

95. Alfredson H, Ohberg L, Forsgren S. Is vasculo-neural ingrowth the cause of pain in chronic Achilles tendinosis? An investigation using ultrasonography and colour Doppler, immunohistochemistry, and diagnostic injections. Knee Surg Sports Traumatol Arthrosc 2003;11(5):334–8.

96. Bjur D, Alfredson H, Forsgren S. The innervation pattern of the human Achilles tendon: studies of the normal and tendinosis tendon with markers for general and sensory innervation. Cell Tissue Res 2005;320(1):201–6.

97. Ljung BO, Alfredson H, Forsgren S. Neurokinin 1-receptors and sensory neuropeptides in tendon insertions at the medial and lateral epicondyles of the humerus. Studies on tennis elbow and medial epicondylalgia. J Orthop Res 2004;22(2):321–7.

98. Ljung BO, Forsgren S, Friden J. Sympathetic and sensory innervations are heterogeneously distributed in relation to the blood vessels at the extensor carpi radialis brevis muscle origin of man. Cells Tissues Organs 1999;165(1):45–54.

99. Guex JJ. Indications for the sclerosing agent polidocanol (aetoxisclerol dexo, aethoxisklerol kreussler). J Dermatol Surg Oncol 1993;19(10):959–61.

100. Hoksrud A, Ohberg L, Alfredson H, et al. Ultrasound-guided sclerosis of neovessels in painful chronic patellar tendinopathy: a randomized controlled trial. Am J Sports Med 2006;34(11):1738–46.

101. Alfredson H, Ohberg L. Sclerosing injections to areas of neo-vascularisation reduce pain in chronic Achilles tendinopathy: a double-blind randomised controlled trial. Knee Surg Sports Traumatol Arthrosc 2005;13(4):338–44.

102. Zeisig E, Fahlstrom M, Ohberg L, et al. Pain relief after intratendinous injections in patients with tennis elbow: results of a randomised study. Br J Sports Med 2008; 42(4):267–71.

103. Tallon C, Coleman BD, Khan KM, et al. Outcome of surgery for chronic Achilles tendinopathy. A critical review. Am J Sports Med 2001;29(3):315–20.

104. Alfredson H, Ohberg L. Neovascularisation in chronic painful patellar tendinosis—promising results after sclerosing neovessels outside the tendon challenge the need for surgery. Knee Surg Sports Traumatol Arthrosc 2005;13(2):74–80.

105. Alfredson H, Harstad H, Haugen S, et al. Sclerosing polidocanol injections to treat chronic painful shoulder impingement syndrome-results of a two-centre collaborative pilot study. Knee Surg Sports Traumatol Arthrosc 2006;14(12):1321–6.

106. Alfredson H, Ohberg L, Zeisig E, et al. Treatment of midportion Achilles tendinosis: similar clinical results with US and CD-guided surgery outside the tendon and sclerosing polidocanol injections. Knee Surg Sports Traumatol Arthrosc 2007; 15(12):1504–9.

107. Clementson M, Loren I, Dahlberg L, et al. Sclerosing injections in midportion Achilles tendinopathy: a retrospective study of 25 patients. Knee Surg Sports Traumatol Arthrosc 2008;16(9):887–90.

108. Knobloch K, Gohritz A, Spies M, et al. Neovascularisation in de Quervain's disease of the wrist: novel combined therapy using sclerosing therapy with polidocanol and eccentric training of the forearms and wrists-a pilot report. Knee Surg Sports Traumatol Arthrosc 2008;16(8):803–5.

109. Lind B, Ohberg L, Alfredson H. Sclerosing polidocanol injections in mid-portion Achilles tendinosis: remaining good clinical results and decreased tendon thickness at 2-year follow-up. Knee Surg Sports Traumatol Arthrosc 2006;14(12):1327–32.

110. Zeisig E, Ohberg L, Alfredson H. Sclerosing polidocanol injections in chronic painful tennis elbow-promising results in a pilot study. Knee Surg Sports Traumatol Arthrosc 2006;14(11):1218–24.

111. Ohberg L, Alfredson H. Sclerosing therapy in chronic Achilles tendon insertional pain-results of a pilot study. Knee Surg Sports Traumatol Arthrosc 2003;11(5): 339–43.

112. Riley GP. Gene expression and matrix turnover in overused and damaged tendons. Scand J Med Sci Sports 2005;15(4):241–51.

113. Vu TH, Werb Z. Matrix metalloproteinases: effectors of development and normal physiology. Genes Dev 2000;14(17):2123–33.

114. Magra M, Maffulli N. Matrix metalloproteases: a role in overuse tendinopathies. Br J Sports Med 2005;39(11):789–91.

115. Clegg PD, Strassburg S, Smith RK. Cell phenotypic variation in normal and damaged tendons. Int J Exp Pathol 2007;88(4):227–35.

116. Orchard J, Massey A, Brown R, et al. Successful management of tendinopathy with injections of the MMP-inhibitor aprotinin. Clin Orthop Relat Res 2008;466(7): 1625–32.

117. Scarpone M, Rabago DP, Zgierska A, et al. The efficacy of prolotherapy for lateral epicondylosis: a pilot study. Clin J Sport Med 2008;18(3):248–54.

118. Banks A. A rationale for prolotherapy. J Orthop Med 1991;13(3):54–9.

119. Rabago D, Best TM, Beamsley M, et al. A systematic review of prolotherapy for chronic musculoskeletal pain. Clin J Sport Med 2005;15(5):376–80.

120. Coombes BK, Bisset L, Vicenzino B. Efficacy and safety of corticosteroid injections and other injections for management of tendinopathy: a systematic review of randomised controlled trials. Lancet 2010;376(9754):1751–67.

121. Spacca G, Necozione S, Cacchio A. Radial shock wave therapy for lateral epicondylitis: a prospective randomised controlled single-blind study. Eura Medicophys 2005;41(1):17–25.

122. Longo UG, Ronga M, Maffulli N. Achilles tendinopathy. Sports Med Arthrosc 2009;17(2):112–26.

123. Kannus P, Jozsa L. Histopathological changes preceding spontaneous rupture of a tendon. A controlled study of 891 patients. J Bone Joint Surg Am 1991;73(10): 1507–25.

124. Paavola M, Kannus P, Jarvinen TA, et al. Treatment of tendon disorders. Is there a role for corticosteroid injection? Foot Ankle Clin 2002;7(3):501–13.

125. Bahr R, Fossan B, Loken S, et al. Surgical treatment compared with eccentric training for patellar tendinopathy (Jumper's Knee). A randomized, controlled trial. J Bone Joint Surg Am 2006;88(8):1689–98.

126. Santander J, Zarba E, Iraporda H, et al. Can arthroscopically assisted treatment of chronic patellar tendinopathy reduce pain and restore function? Clin Orthop Relat Res 2011.[Epub ahead of print].

127. Baker CL Jr, Baker CL 3rd. Long-term follow-up of arthroscopic treatment of lateral epicondylitis. Am J Sports Med 2008;36(2):254–60.

128. Grewal R, MacDermid JC, Shah P, et al. Functional outcome of arthroscopic extensor carpi radialis brevis tendon release in chronic lateral epicondylitis. J Hand Surg Am 2009;34(5):849–57.

129. Lattermann C, Romeo AA, Anbari A, et al. Arthroscopic debridement of the extensor carpi radialis brevis for recalcitrant lateral epicondylitis. J Shoulder Elbow Surg 2010;19(5):651–6.

130. Maffulli N, Testa V, Capasso G, et al. Results of percutaneous longitudinal tenotomy for Achilles tendinopathy in middle- and long-distance runners. Am J Sports Med 1997;25(6):835–40.

131. Testa V, Capasso G, Benazzo F, et al. Management of Achilles tendinopathy by ultrasound-guided percutaneous tenotomy. Med Sci Sports Exerc 2002;34(4): 573–80.
132. van Dijk CN, Kort N, Scholten PE. Tendoscopy of the posterior tibial tendon. Arthroscopy 1997;13(6):692–8.
133. van Dijk CN, van Dyk GE, Scholten PE, et al. Endoscopic calcaneoplasty. Am J Sports Med 2001;29(2):185–9.
134. Scholten PE, van Dijk CN. Endoscopic calcaneoplasty. Foot Ankle Clin 2006;11(2): 439–46, viii.
135. Thermann H, Benetos IS, Panelli C, et al. Endoscopic treatment of chronic mid-portion Achilles tendinopathy: novel technique with short-term results. Knee Surg Sports Traumatol Arthrosc 2009;17(10):1264–9.
136. Maffulli N, Longo UG, Denaro V. Novel approaches for the management of tendi-nopathy. J Bone Joint Surg 2010;92(15):2604–13.

Rehabilitation of Running Injuries

Terry L. Nicola, MD, MS[a,b,c,]*, Amir El Shami, MD[c]

KEYWORDS

- Rehabilitation • Running injuries • Overuse injuries
- Tendinopathy • Stress fracture • Lower limb

Running injuries to the lower extremities are typically caused by cumulative trauma. There are both acute and chronic features to these injuries. To address this prolonged history of recurrent injury, we use a multifaceted plan for treatment and rehabilitation. In guiding treatment, it is important to understand the predisposing factors to the injury. Determining these factors will help guide an individualized treatment plan for the runner, which can include counseling the runner on more effective training and providing specific rehabilitation guidelines once the runner is ready to return to training.

Several determining factors have been associated with injury in runners, including age, body weight, alignment, previous running experience, shoes, running terrain, and even psychological factors. In the evaluation of a runner, one should be evaluating for both intrinsic and extrinsic factors. Underlying intrinsic risk factors include strength and flexibility deficits, which can be applied to the rehabilitation plan. When possible, a thorough evaluation of running gait can clue the clinician in to an inciting cause of injury and help the runner's rehabilitation. Extrinsic factors, as a cause for injury in runners, are often attributed to some alteration in the runner's training, including a change in volume, intensity, distance, footwear, or change in running surfaces.[1,2] Previous running experience can also guide diagnosis and rehabilitation.

INITIAL STRATEGIES

Initial rehabilitation starts by managing inflammation with PRICE: Protection, Rest, Ice, Compression, and Elevation.

The authors have nothing to disclose.
[a] UIC Sports Medicine Center, 839 West Roosevelt Avenue, Suite #102, Chicago, IL 60608, USA
[b] Department of Orthopedic Surgery, University of Illinois at Chicago, Chicago, IL, USA
[c] Family Medicine Department, University of Illinois at Chicago, Chicago, IL, USA
* Corresponding author. UIC Sports Medicine Center, 839 West Roosevelt Avenue, Suite #102, Chicago, IL 60608.
E-mail address: tnicola@uic.edu

Clin Sports Med 31 (2012) 351–372
doi:10.1016/j.csm.2011.10.002
0278-5919/12/$ – see front matter © 2012 Elsevier Inc. All rights reserved.

Protection

Protection involves devices that support the injured tissue to restrict motion or provide cushioning. Protection of the injured area is especially difficult with runners. They resist any reduction in physical activity, especially as it applies to running.

If pain-free weight bearing is not possible through protective bracing, then a course of crutches may be warranted. Efforts to allow limited walking or running activity for mild injuries by some forms of athletic taping may be only tolerated if it is a lo-dye style of tape that helps protect stresses to the foot plantar surface. However, the tape loosens within less than an hour.[3] Foot orthoses may be applied for this same purpose. There is no clear difference in protective effect for over-the-counter and custom foot orthoses for injury prevention in the general population. However, for protection of select patients with uniquely shaped feet, especially in the subacute phases of injury, there may be some benefit to custom-fitted orthoses. However, it is not clear whether these devices should be worn temporarily through the healing phases of injury versus their use in the long term. There are significant concerns about overprotection of feet and overall lower extremity movement from use of restrictive lower extremity devices and footwear.

Further efforts to reduce lower extremity weight bearing, especially with unstable stress fractures[4] of the fifth metatarsal, tarsal bones, sesamoid, anterior midtibia, femoral neck, and pelvis may be necessary for 6 to 12 weeks. Crutch support limited between toe touch and partial weight bearing is determined by the site and acuity of injury as well as indicators of healing, such as callus formation.

Note that shoes may be confining and delay healing, especially if there is swelling. A walking boot may be helpful to reduce stress to the foot and ankle without exacerbating symptoms. Splints in conjunction with crutches may be helpful for Achilles tendinopathy and Achilles tendon ruptures (plantarflexion). Splints also have a unique role for plantar fasciosis. Splinting the ankle at 90° flexion during sleep has been shown to significantly improve morning pain.[5] We have used lace-up ankle braces during the day to support the arch or a more rigid plastic ankle foot orthosis for more severe cases.

Other protective devices, especially at the knee level, such as patellar choker straps, knee sleeves, and more specialized braces, are not proven to help in the early phases of knee injuries, especially to the patellofemoral mechanism.[6] The exception may be knee and ankle swelling as well as hamstring strains treated by compressive sleeves. Calf sleeves can worsen compartment syndrome.

Rest

One of the most challenging aspects of rehabilitating a runner is agreeing on an adequate amount of rest to provide pain relief and recovery. In general, the severity of the injury and pain dictate how quickly a runner can progress back to regular training. Certain fractures are high risk according to their specific location (such as the anterior tibial cortex) and require special treatment. However, for most stress fractures, relative rest from running is the most important initial treatment.[7] If there is pain with ambulation, then crutch walking or a limited period of non–weight bearing is indicated. For soft tissue injuries to the lower extremity, an initial trial of a short or long walking boot may be indicated. More often, cessation of running is all that is necessary to control pain. The rate of activity resumption is dependent on the severity of the injury and the premorbid functional level of the runner. Strategies for return to training will be discussed later in this article. Daily activities should be pain free before return to training. For stress fractures there should be no bony tenderness, and for soft tissue injuries there should be minimal residual tenderness. In general, a period of 1 to 2 weeks of pain-free daily activities should be present before any consideration of return to running. If pain should recur, a short period of rest with resumption of training at a lower level is appropriate.

Ice

Hypothermia has been shown to be effective during the acute phases of inflammation. Cooling of injured tissue decreases blood flow, which is purported to reduce secondary tissue hypoxia from edema.[8] Other potential beneficial effects come from local analgesic effects, decreased muscle spasm, reduced nerve conduction velocity, and reduced metabolic tissue demand. A critical review of treatment for soft tissue injuries of the ankle found a positive benefit of cryotherapy.[9] There are several effective application methods for producing hypothermia, including ice packs, ice massage, cold whirlpool, and cold compression. Despite the leading role of ice in the rehabilitation of acute injuries, little evidence exists to guide which method of cryotherapy is most effective. Nonetheless, alternate modalities are free from the side effects of anti-inflammatory agents. Cold urticaria, and "freezer burn" can be avoided by proper history, trial of a cold pack in office, and avoidance of hypesthetic skin, such as an area of prior skin burn. Cryopalsy of the peroneal nerve from application of cold pack wrap to the knee has been described. This is most likely because of overexposure to freezing temperature or prolonged effects of compression from the knee wrap. Fortunately, this side effect is rare.

We have found ice and water cold packs or frozen vegetables are the most reliable and easiest to use. We recommend applying the ice pack without excessive pressure for 15 to 20 minutes, 2 to 4 times per day as tolerated. For the multiple foot and ankle stresses to the forefoot, plantar fascia, and tendinopathies, ice and water footbath can be very effective. Our written instructions are as follows:

1. Fill a plastic garbage can or deep washbasin with water.
2. Place injured distal lower extremity in the water.
3. Dump ice into the water for cold effect.

This approach to ice water immersion is well tolerated by runners.

Compression

Increased swelling is associated with increased secondary tissue damage and range of motion deficits. For most runners, effective compression can be carried out with a compression stocking with 15 to 20 mmHg of graded pressure. Compression socks are also being used routinely by some runners to prevent edema, and many sports stores are now carrying varying brands and types. Compression of distal lower extremity injuries, especially of the ankle with poor, excessively tight, elastic bandaging can lead to increased distal edema. Careful attention to a climbing Figure 8 wrapping should be used.

Elevation

The injured limb should be placed at least 15 cm above the heart to facilitate venous and lymphatic drainage to prevent build up of edema. Note that leg elevation may be helpful during a midrun break or after a run. Leg swelling may occur from the effects of a long run or after prolonged standing, even when not injured.

The PRICE acronym can also be expanded to PRICEMM to include medications and modalities.

Medications

Nonsteroidal anti-inflammatory drugs (NSAIDs) have not been shown to change the outcome of running injuries. Their use may even cause an increase in inflammatory markers if taken during long distance racing.[10] Nevertheless, sudden onset of swelling from synoviits at the ankle and knee may benefit from short-term improved mobility if NSAIDs reduce the swelling.

For pain relief, NSAIDs, acetaminophen, or other analgesics are commonly used. For acute soft tissue injuries, NSAIDs are generally recommended over other analgesics for their anti-inflammatory properties. For acute fractures, there is increasing evidence that NSAIDs can prolong healing time.[7] However, evidence that NSAIDs impair healing for stress fractures has not been seen. Nonetheless, avoidance of NSAIDs for stress fractures of the lower extremity is still recommended.

Heat

Heat as a modality can be effective for symptomatic relief of chronic muscle injuries but in acute injuries can actually worsen edema and swelling.

ULTRASOUND

Therapeutic ultrasound has been recommended to relieve pain after muscle injury and to enhance the initial stages of muscle regeneration, yet its use does not appear to have a beneficial influence on muscle healing.[11,12]

BONE STIMULATORS

Electrical and electromagnetic bone growth stimulation has been tried for treatment of fractures and stress fractures. Bone stimulators are used frequently for delayed unions and nonunions but are not routinely used for the treatment of acute fractures or stress fractures.[13] There is insufficient evidence to support the use of electromagnetic bone growth stimulation. However the evidence for electrical bone stimulation does trend in favor of its use for achieving bony union.[14] There is some evidence that low-intensity pulsed ultrasonography can improve healing of fresh fractures.[15] Although overall results are promising, the utility in stress fractures is less clear. Establishing the role of low-intensity pulsed ultrasonography in the management of stress fractures will require further investigation.

MASSAGE

For the chronic overuse injuries, there is an association with muscle weakness, loss of flexibility, and tenderness. Massage has been very popular among runners for these signs and symptoms. Self massage can be effective in helping relieve secondary local muscle spasm and hasten recovery. A treatment first popularized by Cyriax in 1978[16] known as cross frictions, can help relieve symptoms associated with chronic muscle injuries. Cross friction performed at the correct pressure by a licensed massage therapist or trained physical therapist is generally uncomfortable and focuses on areas of tender muscle "knots." As chronic muscle injuries tend to recur, cross friction massage at the first sign of reinjury can sustain an athlete's running regimen.

Conflicting evidence exists regarding massage therapy and its positive effect on hamstring muscle activity and flexibility in healthy adults[17–19] with no evidence regarding its effect on healing and recovery after an acute muscle strain injury.

BRACING (SEE PROTECTION)

Bracing can be functional, rehabilitative, or prophylactic in nature. Most leg devices can be detrimental for return to running, as they can add another biomechanical variable to the runner. Initial bracing in a short or long walking boot can help rest injured tissue during the nonrunning phase of rehabilitation. There is concern that one may become weak in a walking boot, and prolonged use can be detrimental. However, judicious bracing with appropriate range of motion and strengthening exercises out of the walking boot can prevent any atrophy or contractures.

TAPING

There is evidence that antipronation tape has a biomechanical effect, demonstrated by increases in navicular height and medial longitudinal arch height, reductions in tibial internal rotation, and calcaneal eversion as well as alteration of plantar pressure patterns, under both static and dynamic conditions.[20]

Augmented low dye taping has been shown recently to significantly increase lateral midfoot plantar pressure and delay the onset of muscle activation patterns during treadmill running.[21] Antipronation taping theoretically decreases the load on muscles that can lead to injury. Electromyographic studies have found diminished activity in the tibialis anterior and tibialis posterior muscles with walking and thus may be helpful in the rehabilitation of injuries involving these muscles.[22]

Other commonly practiced taping techniques in runners include kinesiotaping or McConnell taping. This technique, which requires a trained therapist or other professional for correct application, has been used to treat patellofemoral pain syndrome (PFPS) for more than 20 years, but its effectiveness is still controversial. McConnell taping technique was originally developed to correct altered patellofemoral kinematics and permit participation in normal daily activity.[23] Today there are several techniques to McConnell taping, and proper clinical application requires an understanding of patellar position, orientation, and mobility. Theoretically medializing the patella in someone with PFPS would offload the compressive forces at the lateral patellofemoral joint and decrease pain. McConnell taping has been shown recently to inferiorly shift the patella in patients with PFPS.[24] These patients with altered patellofemoral kinematics are likely to benefit from an inferior shift of the patella, which should reduce patellofemoral contact stresses and thus diminish pain.

INJECTIONS

Injections in acute and subacute running injuries are rarely indicated. One exception is osteitis pubis, which may respond to first-line use of a corticosteroid injection. For more chronic injuries, the number of indications increase. Because running injuries are typically recurrent with both acute inflammatory and chronic noninflammatory features, corticosteroid injections have been delivered as peritenon injections near the Achilles tendon to reduce hypertrophic fibrotic tissue. Similarly, corticosteroid injections have been used for plantar fasciosis (also called plantar fasciitis), although it is not really known what the benefit is from the injection. It is not clear if the pain is addressed because of reduction of fibrotic tissue or if the plantar fascia may atrophy or tear from this injection leading to less stress at the origin. Sites of bursitis have been candidates for injection, such as the distal iliotibial band friction syndrome, greater trochanter, pes anserinus, Baker's cyst, suprapatellar bursa, and iliopsoas bursa.[25] It can be questioned, especially with the increased use of diagnostic ultrasound scan, that the bursitis is a cause for pain. Most of these painful sites under ultrasound scan uncommonly show evidence for a bursitis.[26] Other uses of corticosteroid injections have been for first metatarsal phalangeal joint pain; Morton's neuroma; and tenosynovitis of the tibialis posterior, flexor hallucis longis, and peroneal tendons as well as for knee plica and ankle synovitis. The risk for tendon rupture is a concern, especially for the Achilles and patellar tendons.

Other injections include proliferants, such as dextrose and platelet rich plasma. They propose to help by causing a localized acute inflammatory response leading to a local fibroblastic generation of new collagen tissue. They may help in areas of chronic connective tissues breakdown at tendon insertion sites (Achilles, patellar, posterior tibial), muscle tears (hamstring), and friction (iliotibial, greater trochanter, pes anserine). These injections do not carry the same risk for tendon rupture as corticosteroids. However, their efficacy in the treatment of running-related injuries has not yet been established.

FOOTWEAR

Recognizing bad shoes and shoe assessment and selection can help prevent further injury and expedite rehabilitation. The general anatomy of a running shoe includes an outsole that contacts the running surface, a midsole composed usually of foam, which provides cushioning and support, the upper part of the shoe that secures the foot to the shoe, and the template or last of the shoe, which can be curved, semicurved, straight and board lasted, slip lasted, or combination lasted. In addition, shoes are variable with regard to their weight and stability or motion control they possess. Billions of dollars are spent by shoe manufacturers to market and promote the beneficial effects of their shoe versus their competition. In actuality, very little evidence exists for the benefit of one shoe versus another. Studies have failed to demonstrate decreased rate of injury with expensive shoes versus less expensive shoes.[27]

The widespread belief that flat-footed, overpronating runners need motion-control shoes and that high-arched, underpronating runners will benefit from well-cushioned pairs is not supported by evidence. A review article from 2009 concluded that the current practice of prescribing distance running shoes featuring elevated cushioned heels and pronation control systems tailored to the individual's foot type is not evidence based.[28] The true effects of today's running shoes on the health and performance of distance runners remains largely unknown. Biomechanical studies of runners on treadmills repeatedly have shown that pronation is significantly reduced in runners who wear motion-control shoes, but it is not known whether pronation is really the underlying issue. Few studies have examined whether over- or underpronation contributes to running injuries.

More and more evidence is now showing that our understanding of running mechanics and shoe recommendations were misinformed and even potentially injurious. A study using experienced distance runners gave underpronators cushiony shoes, overpronators motion-control shoes, and the remainder of runners shoes at random.[29] They found no influence on injury even after considering other injury risk factors and even found a majority of injuries occurring in runners with shoes specifically designed for them, and across the board, motion-control shoes were the most injurious.[29] There are probably only a few runners for whom motion-control shoes are appropriate, and extreme caution should be used in prescribing them. A study in military recruits found no correlation between wearing the proper running shoes for their arch type and avoiding injury.[30] The highest injury rates were actually seen among soldiers who received shoes designed specifically for their foot types. It is important to inform runners that there is no one shoe superior to the others. There is no break-in period for running shoes, and if they do not feel good immediately, they are not for you. Also, even if a runner has used a particular brand or model for some time, each and every shoe can have a different feel, fit, and flexibility. We recommend looking for the lightest shoe possible that feels good and holds the patient up (ie, in single leg stance the shoe holds the foot upright without collapsing in too far).

STRENGTHENING

Core strengthening is often neglected in runners. More recently, the emphasis and understanding of a strong core on running has come to fruition. In the rehabilitation of an injured runner, an assessment of core strength and a rehabilitation program addressing it can help the rehabilitation, reduce further injury, and even improve the efficiency of running. For example, in the pelvic core, weakness leads to malalignment of the pelvis, which can be transmitted into the lower extremities predisposing the runner to hamstring injuries and Achilles problems. A stronger core also improves the body's stability when it contacts the ground, reducing unnecessary stabilization and overuse injury from other parts of the body. Also increased stabilization on landing is more economical to the runner and can lead to better times.

FLEXIBILITY

Flexibility training must be approached within a program aimed at addressing the specific functional needs of the individual. The most common flexibility issues contributing to injuries in runners include the iliotibial band, hamstring, hip flexors, and gastrocsoleus complex. Changes in flexibility immediately after instituting a stretching program are attributed to neural factors, and thus an early flexibility program can provide significant benefit in runners. Further changes in flexibility require a change in sarcomere number to establish a new structural muscle length and can take several months to become apparent.[31,32] Techniques available for improving flexibility include static, passive, and proprioceptive neuromuscular facilitation.

Static stretching, defined as elongation of a muscle to tolerance and applying a steady force for a length of time,[33,34] is considered the easiest, most popular and safest form of stretching. Passive stretching incorporates a slow and sensitive application of force by a partner or therapist who applies a stretch to a relaxed joint or extremity. Proprioceptive neuromuscular facilitation (PNF) is a method of stretching combing static stretching and isometric contractions to improve flexibility and coordination through a limb's entire range of motion. More recently, advocated methods include dynamic stretching or improving flexibility by eccentrically training a muscle through its full range of motion.

Questions abound regarding the utility of static stretching to reduce injuries or improve athletic performance.[35–37] Studies have not shown static stretching to reduce injury rates.[38–40] and pre competition stretching may actually be a detriment to performance.[41]

Dynamic flexibility involves contracting the antagonist muscle group, thus allowing the agonist to elongate naturally in a relaxed state.[42] An exercise we recommend often that utilizes this principle is called "knee press with fighting feet." For this exercise, a rolled up towel is placed behind the knee, and the knee is pressed down while simultaneously opposing dorsiflexion with the heel of the opposite foot (**Figs. 1** and **2**). This is accompanied by active contract and relax exercises of the quadriceps, which stretch the hamstrings as well. Theoretically, the dynamic nature of the stretch will cause increased neural level activation of the affected muscle, accommodating the stretch and increasing flexibility. Training a

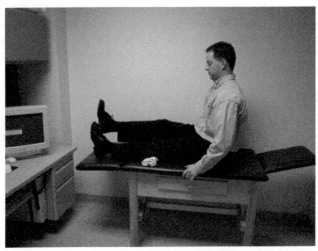

Fig. 1. Rehabilitation of running injuries. Patellofemoral: knee press with fighting feet.

muscle incorporating the largest muscle tendon loads through its full range of motion would theoretically improve flexibility and reduce injury rate. Training a muscle through a full range of motion will improve flexibility over a period of 6 weeks as well as static stretching. A recent study found an immediate benefit on hamstring flexibility using eccentric training of a muscle through its full range of motion with use of the antagonist muscle over static stretching methods. These subjects had tight hamstring pretreatment, but it is unknown if there is benefit to the injured running population, and further investigation is warranted.

BALANCE

Each step taken while running is a single leg stance, and balance training is the neuromuscular link allowing runners to improve this control. Balance training integrates

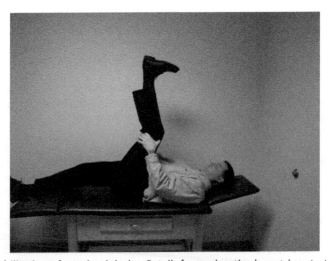

Fig. 2. Rehabilitation of running injuries. Patellofemoral: active hamstring stretch.

core strengthening, lower body strengthening, flexibility, and muscle mobility. Proprioception refers to a sense of joint position and is common in rehabilitation of injured runners and to prevent injury. Slight deviations in terrain while running require slight adjustments of balance to avoid injury. Particular injuries, especially to the foot, can lead to balance deficits and weakness of the foot intrinsic musculature. Continued or recurrent injury may be caused by inadequate balance and proprioceptive rehabilitation. Balance training aids come in a variety of forms such as a balance pad or BOSU ball, although one can just as easily improve their balance with simple exercises such as the one leg squat and reach.

MAINTENANCE OF FITNESS—CROSS TRAINING

Maintaining fitness during treatment of lower-limb injuries is of significant concern to the running athlete. Cross training can maintain fitness with little stress to an injured lower extremity. Cross training is also a useful training adjunct in the noninjured runner for overall fitness and prevention of injury.

Non–weight-bearing methods to maintain cardiovascular fitness include cycling, swimming, deepwater running, and gravity-eliminated running. For most runners, cycling and swimming can be adequate to maintain aerobic fitness without undue stress to the underlying injury. However, for the competitive runner, it is important to abide by the principle of sport specificity to maintain appropriate neuromuscular recruitment patterns. Deep-water running with a flotation device is an effective form of cross-training for the injured runner.[17] During 4- to 8-week deepwater run training programs, runners maintained Vo_2max, anaerobic threshold, leg strength, and 2-mile and 5K run performance.[43]

RUNNING SKILLS AND DRILLS

In the running world, there is a lot of discussion about pronation and supination. However, keep in mind that these are normal motions associated with running. Most runners heel strike laterally, then the heel undergoes normal pronation as the body moves over the planted foot. As the weight of the body is transferred through the midfoot, the foot undergoes supination until toe push off. Alterations in this pattern that are clinically important can be very subtle. This is where inspection of wear patterns on running shoes can be helpful. Based on the normal running motion, increased wear typically occurs over the lateral heel. Overpronation may be present if the mid or medial heel shoe increased wear. Similarly, if a lateral heel wear pattern and wear over the lateral forefoot is present, then underpronation may be present.

In the assessment of running gait, we look for symmetry, completeness of stride, and straight, upright posture. We incorporate various drills during our assessment to help the runner address any issues we see. To encourage an upright running posture, we have the runner place their hands on their hips, followed by hands behind head, and finally followed by reaching up overhead, all while running. Incorporating these drills periodically will encourage the runner to assume a more efficient "tall" running posture. To help the runner complete their stride, we have he or she complete a high, exaggerated forward leg kick.

RETURN TO RUNNING

Various recommendations have been suggested for returning runners to sport after injury. One approach advocates beginning with slow running for one-third of the usual distance alternating with a rest day after symptoms have significantly subsided. If the runner is pain free over the next 2 weeks, he or she may advance weekly mileage and

Table 1 Novice/Intermediate return to running program: Walk-to-run program (cyclic pattern)				
Level[a]	Walk	Run	Distance (miles)	Miles/Week[b]
1	3 min	30 sec	2–3	6–8
2	3 min	1 min	2–3	8–10
3	2 min	1 min	2–4	8–12
4	2 min	2 min	2–5	8–12
5	1 min	3 min	3–5	10–14
6	1 min	5 min	3–6	10–14
7	1 min	Mile	3–6	10–14

Do not run until you are able to walk comfortably at 4.0 mph for 10 miles per week.
[a] Each level usually represents a week.
[b] Miles per week may be more depending on runner ability and baseline endurance.

slowly increase speed and intensity. Rest days should be continued for at least 4 weeks, and cross-training should be incorporated whenever possible.[44,45]

At our clinic, we like to begin weight-bearing exercise with uphill treadmill walking. We recommend walking at 3 to 4 mph at an incline as high as possible that the runner can tolerate for a time that they would normally run. This low-impact, weight-bearing activity will begin to condition the runner's legs to help them transition back into a running program with greater ease and success.

Depending on the runner's experience, we initiate 1 of 2 walk-to-run programs. The experienced program allows the patient to start at a higher level and return to full running sooner. An example of our 2 recommended programs are seen in **Tables 1** and **2**. The Borg Rating of Perceived Exertion 6 to 20 scale is used for more experienced runners. We prefer to use perceived effort to help the experienced runners control their pace without overtraining.[46]

Both walk-to-run programs begin at half the total weekly mileage before the injury occurred. Also they follow the 10% rule that states that a runner should never increase their weekly mileage by more than 10% over the previous week or month.

The association between risk of injury and increasing weekly mileage has been known for some time.[47,48] Reducing weekly mileage is continually shown to be a factor in preventing running injuries; however, no strong evidence exists with regard

Table 2 Experienced return to running program: Walk-to-run program (cyclic pattern)
• You can try walking on incline as tolerated at 3.5–4.0 mph for time you would have run as the initial test for running—2 weeks.
• Return to running should be based on effort. Walk whenever your (Borg 6–20 scale) effort is greater than 14 out of 20.
• Running must be at greater than 5.5 mph. If fatigue or effort is greater than 14 out of 20, then walk. Avoid foot ground scraping.
• Start half of previous weekly mileage. Add 10% per week, increase in mileage, as tolerated without fatigue or pain.[a]
• Do not run until you are able to walk comfortably at 4.0 mph for 10 miles per week.

[a] Miles per week may be more depending on runner ability and baseline endurance.

to proven methods of safely increasing weekly mileage.[49] Weekly mileage has shown significant positive correlations with patellofemoral force and etiology of iliotibial band friction syndrome.[50,51]

SPECIFIC INJURIES
Plantar Fasciitis

Rehabilitating plantar fasciitis can take several months depending on its severity and duration. We recommend an aggressive multifaceted rehabilitation program for plantar fasciitis that involves initial cessation of running and other weight-bearing exercises including walking and elliptical training. If there is significant pain with walking, then an initial trial up to 5 weeks in a walking boot is warranted. We provide runners with a list of instructions, referred to as a *plantar fascia program*.

1. Frequent ice water foot baths
2. Golf ball massage to fleshy part of foot. Avoid direct pressure over heel.
3. Calf raises
4. Maintenance of fitness with stationary bicycling, swimming, or running in water
5. Night splinting.

An anterior night splint to maintain the foot at 90° has been shown to be effective both short term and long term in treating pain from plantar fasciitis.[5] We utilize a lace-up ankle brace to provide this function and find they are more comfortable and tolerated by patients. Principles of strengthening and flexibility as applied to the rehabilitation of Achilles tendonosis apply here as well. We also institute barefoot calf raises beginning with both feet supported, progressing to alternating, "bicycle" calf raises and finally to single leg calf raises. No more than 2 sets of 10 repetitions are initially needed, and the patient can progress based on symptoms. We strongly encourage maintenance of fitness with swimming, running in the water, or stationary bicycling if they can do it without pain. Daily shoe wear is scrutinized with emphasis on well-fitting shoes with good long arch support to take pressure off of the plantar fascia. Often, we recommend a Hapad or even simple gauze and tape for added long and transverse arch support. For recalcitrant pain we consider an ultrasound-guided plantar fascia origin prolotherapy injection. A corticosteroid injection of the plantar fascia origin is often utilized. Although there is often short-term relief of symptoms, there does not appear to be evidence for any long-term benefit.[52,53] If a patient is progressing very slowly or not at all, we recommend a custom molded plastic ankle foot orthosis for a period of 6 to 8 weeks. Once a patient has minimal to no morning pain, we begin a conditioning program of uphill treadmill walking. This weight-bearing exercise has decreased heel strike compared with level ground walking and can be undertaken at a high cardiovascular load with minimal increased pressure to the heel and plantar fascia. This will help condition the runner's legs for a return to running via a walk-to-run program. Magnetic resonance imaging of the ankle can be useful in some cases of plantar fasciitis to rule out concomitant pathology and to determine the amount of associated calcaneal edema surrounding the origin of the plantar fascia, which we have found to somewhat correlate with the need for more rigid ankle foot orthosis protection of the heel.

Foot

Common injuries of the foot in runners include posterior tibialis and flexor hallucis longus tendinopathy and hallux valgus (bunion deformity). Often the most important aspect of rehabilitation for these injuries is proper shoe wear or orthotic use. For hallux valgus with bunion deformity, running shoes with a wider forefoot often is

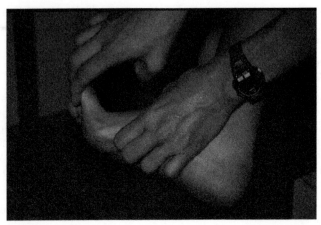

Fig. 3. Rehabilitation of running injuries. Great toe and flexor hallucis longis stretch.

needed to relieve pressure off of the bunion. We have found that daily stretching of the hallux can be helpful and even improve the angle of the hallux valgus. This is accomplished by placing one hand on the foot plantar surface while the other gently distracts then extends and flexes the great the toe with the other hand rhythmically for about 10 repetitions (**Fig. 3**). Surgery often is felt to be the definitive treatment for bunions; however, a randomized, controlled trial showed no differences in health-related quality-of-life score at 1 year between a surgical, orthotic, or watchful waiting group.[54] A follow-up study found the least intense pain in surgical group at 1 year but similar pain intensity in all 3 groups at 2 years.[55]

For flexor hallucis longus (FHL) tendinopathy, Conservative treatment includes decreased activity, passive stretching of the great toe, and changes in shoe wear that allow room for the great toe. Daily rocker bottom type shoes can effectively brace and rest the FHL tendon during regular daily activities.

Posterior tibialis tendon injuries can be rehabilitated initially using conservative methods with emphasis on shoes, orthotics, or taping to control excess pronation and increased tendon strain and to allow more efficient muscle function. For more severe injuries, a period of up to 8 weeks of immobilization with the foot in inversion or in a walking boot with added medial longitudinal arch support may be needed.

Ankle Sprains

Running on uneven surfaces or biomechanical imbalances in the foot can lead to ankle sprains in runners, and rehabilitation for runners follows the same principles as those of other athletes. Treatment for all lateral ankle sprains is conservative with PRICE followed by a functional ankle balance program with early mobilization. The runner should initially refrain from activities that exacerbate the pain and the immediate use of crutches to allow achievement of pain-free weight bearing may be considered. Significant swelling is often seen after lateral ankle sprains and is related to loss of range of motion of the ankle joint. Hence, edema management is key to successful rehabilitation, and this can be accomplished via elastic bandage wrapping or by our preferred method of a compression stocking at 15 to 20 mmHg pressure.

Early mobilization is preferential, and minimizing immobilization has been shown to hasten recovery time.[56,57] Immediate functional rehabilitation will help to stimulate stronger and better-oriented collagen replacement fibers.[58] The progression of a functional rehabilitation program should be regaining range of motion, progressive strengthening exercises, proprioceptive training, and finally running-specific training. Range of motion should initially involve stretching the Achilles tendon to prevent tissue contraction. This can be accomplished without weight bearing using a towel to passively pull the toes or weight bearing with standing knee bends. Another commonly used method is drawing of the alphabet with the foot several times a day.[59] Once pain and swelling are controlled, and range of motion is maintained, progression to strengthening begins. All 4 directions of ankle movement are utilized to strengthen weakened muscles, especially the peroneals in a lateral ankle injury.[58,60] We begin with dynamic resistance bands and encourage pain-free, controlled movement. Emphasis is placed on the eccentric component of the exercise with a 4/1 ratio of eccentric to concentric contraction. Three sets of 10 repetitions completed twice daily are recommended.[60] Commonly utilized exercises in physical therapy include toe curls and marble pick ups, which can also be helpful. Finally, and perhaps most importantly, is proprioceptive rehabilitation. Proprioceptive deficits can lead to repeated ankle injuries. Various devices can help accomplish this, such as a balance pad or balance ball. If a runner does not have access to this equipment, we recommend simply a pillow placed on a hard surface to produce some instability to help with balance exercises. Single-leg balance exercises are recommended once good double leg balance has been attained.

Achilles Tendinopathy and Enthesopathy

Treatment of Achilles tendinopathy or enthesopathy can be difficult and prolonged, often requiring a significant period of rest from running to return without pain. Achilles enthesopathy, or pain at the insertion site, is more frequently seen in jumping and sprinting sports than in long distance running.

For insertional Achilles enthesopathy, if the runner has pain with walking, then a course of immobilization in a walking boot for 4 to 6 weeks should be implemented. As always, maintenance of cardiovascular fitness is important for eventual return to running and often for runner sanity with bicycling, swimming, or running in the water. Excess calcaneal valgus can precipitate pain and injury to the Achilles insertion and should be corrected with heel/arch lifts or orthoses. Achilles stretching should be implemented early followed by an eccentric loading program. However, the response rate in enthesopathy is reported to be much less than that of midportion Achilles tendinopathy. For runners that continue to have pain and functional difficulties with enthesopathy despite these interventions, we recommend an ultrasound-guided percutaneous tenotomy using a proliferative mixture of 50% dextrose and 1% lidocaine. After prenumbing the area with lidocaine, we identify, under ultrasound, cortical irregularities on the calcaneus at the Achilles insertion. Using a 21-gauge needle, we attempt to break up the irregularities and stimulate inflammation with repeated needling and injection of the proliferants. This same procedure is also being utilized using platelet-rich plasma in place of the proliferant.[61]

For midportion Achilles tendinopathy, initial treatment includes cessation of running, avoidance of hill running, and Achilles stretching. Hyperpronation should be corrected with orthotics. Even a neutral foot will benefit from medial longitudinal arch support to decrease strain on the Achilles tendon. If no rupture is seen on imaging, then an eccentric exercise program should be instituted. Several studies have documented the benefit of an eccentric exercise program for noninsertional Achilles tendinopathy. The preferred method involves standing on a step with the ankle neutral and then slowly lowering the heel to maximum ankle dorsiflexion. We recommend doing these exercises barefoot starting with both legs, followed by alternating "bicycle" leg and then single leg. Also doing the exercises with a flexed knee will preferentially activate the soleus. Recommendations of how many sets and repetitions of exercises can be up to 3 sets of 15 repetitions 3 times weekly with the knee flexed and knee extended. Patients should expect to have some increased pain initially, but this should subside over the course of 1 to 2 weeks.

If diagnostic ultrasound scan does not show tearing or partial rupturing of the tendon, and there is hypertrophic tendinosis, we consider a peritenon corticosteroid injection. Certainly, corticosteroid injection directly into the tendon has been associated with complete rupture and is discouraged. Ill-fitting shoes with increased pressure and rubbing of the posterior calcaneus and Achilles tendon should be addressed. We actually cut a vertical incision into the posterior part of the shoe to expand the heel and secure with tape to accommodate the Achilles tendon.

Plica and Patellofemoral Syndrome

Often these 2 injuries will coexist or complicate one another, and treatment of one should include treatment of the other. For an inflamed, symptomatic plica, aggressive icing with ice cube massage or a frozen Dixie cup is utilized in combination with a simple medial patella stretch. The stretch can be performed easily by the runner cupping the superior portion of the patella and applying gentle medial inferior pressure, holding for a bout 30 seconds and repeating as frequently as possible. Several biomechanical factors may be contributing to the development of PFPS, including weak hip and pelvic rotators, a tight iliotibial band, tight hamstrings, weak quadriceps especially the vastus medialis oblique, wide Q angle, a leg length discrepancy, and overpronating feet. It is not clear which of these factors may be most important in the development of PFPS, but any of these identified factors should be addressed for a successful rehabilitation. Again, an initial period of rest can be very helpful for the successful rehabilitation of PFPS. Despite the uncertainty, it does appear that a majority of PFPS will respond favorably to an eccentric quadriceps strengthening program using wall slides or single leg squat exercises. Improving iliotibial band flexibility with foam rolling and stretching is helpful.[62] If a runner has significant pes plano valgum (or overpronating feet contributing to genu valgum) and a lateral tracking patella, then we recommend a foot orthosis with medial arch support to bring them into a more neutral position.[6] Another approach to treating PFPS focuses more on proximal strengthening about the hip.[63] Here it is felt that it is not so much an abnormally laterally tracking patella caused by weak quadriceps or a tight iliotibial band as the cause of the injury, but rather weak proximal hip muscles. Specifically, the hip rotators and abductors fail to control femoral motion, properly causing it to rotate abnormally and create contact between the femoral condyles and the posterior patella, generating pain.[63] Therefore, a program of proximal hip strengthening can improve symptoms. We recommend a physical therapy program addressing both of these areas. To maintain fitness, swimming or running in the water is recommended. Bicycling can sometimes aggravate PFPS, but if a runner can bicycle without reproduction of symptoms, then we encourage it. It is important to have the seat as high as possible to limit the amount of knee flexion with pedaling.

Popliteus Strain

This uncommon injury can be quite debilitating to a runner, and principles of rehabilitation follow those of other muscular tendinopathies. The popliteus can become tight in spasm when there is poor hamstring or quadriceps strength; thus, rehabilitation should focus on eccentric strengthening of these muscle groups.

Nyland and coworkers[64] described a set of 3 exercises for popliteus tendinopathy involving an isolated strengthening exercise, a loading-unloading step exercise, and a stepping task performed on an unstable surface. The isolated strengthening exercise consists of securing a resistance band to the forefoot of the affected leg. The affected leg is then brought behind the stance leg via external rotation of the hip and knee flexion, and the affected leg continues behind the stance leg with increasing internal tibial rotation. The return to neutral provides an eccentric muscle effort. A dynamic stepping exercise utilizes the following routine: the affected leg is brought posterior and lateral to stance leg, far forward, posterior, and medial to stance leg, far forward again, then finally far sideward of the stance leg. This exercise can then be completed with the stance leg on an unstable surface.

Iliotibial Band Syndrome

Activity modification with no running is recommended based on symptoms. Alternative activities such as deep water running or swimming should be encouraged. Repetitive flexion activities such as bicycling often can also reproduce symptoms in running-induced iliotibial band syndrome (ITBS) and should initially be discouraged. As symptoms allow, long walks (30 minutes or longer depending on runner's history of training) should be followed by inclined treadmill walking (incline as tolerated) for the same amount of time. If asymptomatic, then a walk-to-run program is the next step. A conservative approach of ice and NSAIDs is helpful for pain control. The emphasis of rehabilitation for ITBS is for an aggressive stretching and massage program to the ITB. A commonly performed ITB stretch involves crossing the affected leg behind you and then leaning toward the contralateral side. One study found that a comprehensive stretching protocol incorporating an overhead arm extension into this commonly performed standing ITB stretch significantly increased ITB flexibility.[65] Aggressive massage and foam rolling of the ITB helps to further increase ITB fascial length. Improving strength of pelvic core (gluteal) muscles and of the quadriceps and hamstrings is needed to stabilize the lower extremity and reduce ITB strain. Strengthening the lateral stabilizers to decrease pelvic tilt is especially important in proximal ITB syndrome. Typical recovery time is 4 to 6 weeks depending on age, fitness, and previous injury level.[66] In refractory cases, a corticosteroid injection into the ITB bursa may significantly improve symptoms and help progression of the rehabilitation program. We advise using a lateral approach under ultrasound guidance to better identify the ITB bursa.

Hamstring Injuries

The primary goal of a hamstring rehabilitation program is to return the runner to their prior level of speed, distance, and performance while minimizing the risk of injury recurrence. An effective rehabilitation program needs to properly address pain, muscular weakness, flexibility deficits, or altered movement patterns associated with the injury. Rehabilitation should involve aspects of soft-tissue mobilization, stretching, and progressive eccentric hamstring strengthening and core stabilization exercises. There is no consensus to the optimal rehabilitation of hamstring injuries. Common aspects of most rehabilitation programs include a stepwise approach with rest, ice, and compression followed by isometric, isotonic, and isokinetic strengthening, then light jogging. Running-related hamstring strain injuries typically occur along an intramuscular tendon or aponeurosis and the adjacent muscle fibers.[67,68] During its recovery from injury, the hamstrings must be rehabilitated properly to safely handle high eccentric loading upon return to running.

Focusing on muscle remodeling, eccentric strength training has been advocated in the rehabilitation of hamstring injuries. The performance of controlled eccentric strength training exercises has been shown to facilitate a shift in peak force development to longer musculotendon length.[69] A common criticism of this type of eccentric strength training is the lack of attention to adjacent musculature. Neuromuscular control of the lumbopelvic region is now recognized to enable optimal function of the hamstrings during running and other normal sporting activities.[70] Hamstring rehabilitation should utilize trunk stabilization and progressive agility exercises.[71,72] For acute hamstring injury, significantly reduced recurrence rates are possible using a progressive agility and trunk stabilization program.[71]

Flexibility deficits often are present around the knee and hip and should be addressed through dynamic flexibility, although its importance on recovery or injury prevention remains unclear.[73,74] Mild hamstring injuries often do not require complete cessation of running, but alteration to a shorter stride may enable the runner to continue running while they rehabilitate the injury.

In recalcitrant cases, corticosteroid injections into the tendon sheath can be helpful. In a study of National Football League players with hamstring strains treated with intramuscular corticosteroid injection, 84% returned to play without missing a game.[75] Eccentric training through a full range of motion improved hamstring flexibility better than static stretching.[76]

Osteitis Pubis

Osteitis pubis is felt to be a self-limited condition; however, even with adequate conservative program of rest, ice, therapeutic modalities, flexibility, and strengthening, it can have a very protracted course of several months.[77,78] Often, a correctable underlying biomechanical issue is responsible for this injury, and an adequate evaluation, including leg lengths, is vital to prescribing effective rehabilitation and orthoses. Corticosteroids often are utilized to hasten recovery and have the most success if utilized within 2 weeks of symptom inception.[79] One case series described the use of dextrose prolotherapy as an effective treatment modality for chronic cases in male kicking sport athletes.[80] We recommend an initial 4- to 8-week course of conservative measures, physical therapy, therapeutic modalities, and biomechanical assessment. If the patient is unable to return to running after this, then we proceed with an ultrasound-guided corticosteroid injection.

Hip Flexor Strain

Iliopsoas strains are commonly seen with passive hyperextension injuries and uphill running.[81] Judicious gluteus medius strengthening exercises should be instituted that do not cause excess strain on the iliopsoas. A recent study found that hip clam exercises with neutral hips cause increased activity of the iliopsoas and can exacerbate a hip flexor tendonitis.[82] Repetitive snapping of the iliopsoas tendon in a runner can lead to pain and development of iliopsoas bursitis. Continued running, walking, or bicycling can exacerbate the pain, and a period of rest may be needed. Effective stretching of the iliopsoas is helpful and often will require the assistance of a therapist. In cases of a true iliopsoas bursitis, an ultrasound-guided corticosteroid injection can be helpful for a quicker resolution of pain and return to running.

Stress Fractures

In general, the severity of the fracture and pain dictate how quickly a runner can progress back to regular training.[4] For most stress fractures, cessation of running is

Table 3 Duration of crutch use for selected stress fractures of the lower extremity	
Stress Fracture Location	Recommended Length of Time for Toe-Touch Weight Bearing
Femoral neck	6 to 8 weeks or until pain free weight bearing
Anterior cortex, midshaft tibia	8 to 12 weeks
Navicular	6 weeks in short leg cast with additional 2 weeks if clinical tenderness still present
Proximal fifth metatarsal	6 to 8 weeks in short leg cast with up to additional 4 weeks if clinical tenderness still present
Sesamoid	6 weeks in short leg cast
Medial malleolus	Until pain free with ambulation, followed by 6 weeks in an pneumatic leg brace (Aircast)

first and foremost. If there is pain with ambulation, then crutch walking or a limited period of non–weight bearing is indicated. If there is a previous history of stress fracture or the fracture is of cancellous bone, a bone mineral density (BMD) assessment is indicated. If low bone density is present, appropriate treatment of negative energy balance, nutritional issues, or metabolic bone disease are necessary (**Table 3**).

Although most stress fractures will heal without complication in a short time, certain high-risk fractures require specific additional treatment, according to the specific fracture location.

High-risk stress fractures, such as femoral neck, anterior tibia, navicular, proximal fifth metatarsal, and sesamoid, require careful protection and weight-bearing restrictions. Other low-risk fractures, such as fibula or calcaneal stress fractures, will require immobilization and rest based on symptoms but usually for 6 weeks, as this is the time it takes bone callus to mature. Prevention of deconditioning in the affected limb is important during a period of rest for stress fractures; however, for some fractures, this will not be possible without pain or increased stress to the injury.

Calf Injuries

In runners, calf injuries can generally be delineated into medial tibial stress syndrome (MTSS), compartment syndrome, or gastrocnemius strains. A period of rest or decrease in intensity can be curative. The treatment of MTSS has been examined in 3 randomized, controlled studies showing rest to be equal to any intervention.[83] Recommendations with regard to continued running are based on symptoms.[84] An initial treatment for runners with MTSS may include off-the-shelf orthotics and calf stretching. However, this regimen should be only 1 component of an individualized rehabilitation program. Several parameters have been investigated as risk factors, and prognostic indicators for MTSS with navicular drop showing correlations the most often.[85,86] Other factors that should be addressed in a rehabilitation program for MTSS are increases in external and internal hip range of motion.[83] We recommend symptom-based activity with medial longitudinal arch support in conjunction with lower leg strengthening, flexibility, and core exercises.

Rehabilitation for compartment syndrome includes addressing all identifiable and modifiable intrinsic and extrinsic risk factors including training surfaces, shoes, training intensity, muscle imbalances, flexibility, and limb alignment. Often after addressing these risk factors, runners will continue to be symptomatic, and unless they can refrain from symptom-inducing activities, surgical referral will be necessary. Attempting to continue running through exertional compartment syndrome is dangerous and can lead to an irreversible acute compartment syndrome and significant functional deficits.

SUMMARY

Rehabilitating the injured runner involves a thorough evaluation of the runner. The running history is at least as critical as the physical examination to determine the risk factors for injury and goals for rehabilitation. The medical assessment should include an office situation in which the runner can be seen walking and running to ensure that the rehabilitation program is complete and successful.

REFERENCES

1. Ekenman I, Hassmen P, Koivula N, et al. Stress fractures of the tibia: can personality traits help us detect the injury-prone athlete? Scand J Med Sci Sports 2001;11:87–95.
2. van Gent RN, Siem D, van Middelkoop M, et al. Incidence and determinants of lower extremity running injuries in long distance runners: a systematic review. Br J Sports Med 2007;41:469–80.
3. Viljakka T. Mechanics of knee and ankle bandages. Acta Orthop Scand 1986;57(1): 54–8.
4. Harrast MA, Colonno D. Stress fractures in runners. Clin Sports Med 2010;29(3):399–416.
5. Roos E, Engström M, Söderberg B. Foot orthoses for the treatment of plantar fasciitis. Foot Ankle Int 2006;27(8):606–11.
6. Fredericson M. Patello femoral pain. In: O'Connor FG, Wilder RP, editors. Textbook of running medicine. 1st edition. New York (NY): McGraw-Hill; 2001. p.169–79.
7. Brukner PD, Bennell KL. Stress fractures. In: O'Connor FG, Wilder RP, editors. Textbook of running medicine. 1st edition. New York (NY): McGraw-Hill; 2001. p. 227–56.
8. Basford JR. Physical Agents. In: Textbook of Running Medicine. New York: McGraw-Hill; 2001. p. 535–56
9. Ogilvie-Harris DJ, Gilbart M. Treatment modalities for soft tissue injuries of the ankle: a critical review. Clin J Sport Med 1995;5(3):175–86.
10. McAnulty SR, Owens JT, McAnulty LS, et al. Ibuprofen use during extreme exercise: effects on oxidative stress and PGE2. Med Sci Sports Exerc 2007;39(7):1075–9.
11. Rantanen J, Thorsson O, Wollmer P, et al. Effects of therapeutic ultrasound on the regeneration of skeletal myofibers after experimental muscle injury. Am J Sports Med 1999;27:54–9.
12. Markert CD, Merrick MA, Kirby TE, et al. Nonthermal ultrasound and exercise in skeletal muscle regeneration. Arch Phys Med Rehabil 2005;86:1304–10.
13. Zura RD, Sasser B, Sabesan V, et al. A survey of orthopaedic traumatologists concerning the use of bone growth stimulators. J Surg Orthop Adv 2007;16(1):1–4.
14. Goldstein C, Sprague S, Petrisor BA. Electrical stimulation for fracture healing: current evidence. J Orthop Trauma 2010;24(Suppl 1):S62–5.
15. Busse JW, Kaur J, Mollon B, et al. Low intensity pulsed ultrasonography for fractures: systematic review of randomized controlled trials. BMJ 2009;338:b351.
16. Cyriax J. Dural pain. Lancet 1978;1(8070):919–21.
17. Bushman BA, Flynn MG, Andres FF, et al. Effect of 4 wk of deep water run training on performance. Med Sci Sports Exerc 1997;29(5):694–9.

18. Barlow A, Clarke R, Johnson N, et al. Effect of massage of the hamstring muscles on selected electromyographic characteristics of biceps femoris during sub-maximal isometric contraction. Int J Sports Med 2007;28:253–6.

19. Hopper D, Deacon S, Das S, et al. Dynamic soft tissue mobilization increases hamstring flexibility in healthy male subjects. Br J Sports Med 2005;39:594–8.

20. Franettovich M, Chapman A, Blanch P, et al. A physiological and psychological basis for anti-pronation taping from a critical review of the literature. Sports Med 2008;38(8): 617–31.

21. Kelly LA, Racinais S, Tanner CM, et al. Augmented low dye taping changes muscle activation patterns and plantar pressure during treadmill running. J Orthop Sports Phys Ther 2010;40(10):648–55.

22. Franettovich M, Chapman A, Vicenzino B. Tape that increases medial longitudinal arch height also reduces leg muscle activity: a preliminary study. Med Sci Sports Exerc 2008;40(4):593–600.

23. McConnell J. The management of chondromalacia patellae: a long term solution. Aust J Physiother 1986;32:215–23.

24. Derasari A, Brindle TJ, Alter KE, et al. McConnell taping shifts the patella inferiorly in patients with patellofemoral pain: a dynamic magnetic resonance imaging study. Phys Ther 2010;90(3):411–9.

25. Howard TM, Rassner LH. Therapeutic and diagnostic injections and aspirations. In: Seidenberg PH, Anthony IB, editors. The sports medicine resource manual. Philadelphia: Saunders; 2008. p. 574–97.

26. Biachi S, Martinoli C, Abdelwahab IF, et al, editors. Ultrasound of the musculoskeletal system. New York: Springer Heidelberg; 2007.

27. Robbins S, Waked E. Hazard of deceptive advertising of athletic footwear. Br J Sports Med 1997;31(4):299–303.

28. Richards CE, Magin PJ, Callister R. Is your prescription of distance running shoes evidence-based? Br J Sports Med 2009;43(3):159–62.

29. Ryan MB, Valiant GA, McDonald K, et al. The effect of three different levels of footwear stability on pain outcomes in women runners: a randomized control trial. Br J Sports Med 2011;45(9):715–21.

30. Knapik JJ, Trone DW, Swedler DI, et al. Injury reduction effectiveness of assigning running shoes based on plantar shape in Marine Corps basic training. Am J Sports Med 2010;38(9):1759–67.

31. Saal J. Flexibility training. In: Kibler W. editor. Functional rehabilitation of sports and musculoskeletal injuries. Gaithersburg (MD): Aspen; 1998. p. 85–97.

32. Shellock FG, Prentice WE. Warming-up and stretching for improved physical performance and prevention of sports-related injuries. Sports Med 1985;2:267–78.

33. Anderson B, Burke ER. Scientific medical and practical aspects of stretching. Clin Sports Med 1991;10:63–87.

34. Iashvili AV. Active and passive flexibility in athletes specializing in different sports. Teorig Praktika Fizicheskoi Kultury 1987;7:51–2.

35. Bandy WD, Irion JM, Briggler M. The effect of time and frequency of static stretching on flexibility of the hamstring muscles. Phys Ther 1997;77:1090–6.

36. Halbertsma JP, VanBolhuis AI, Goeken LN. Sport stretching: effect on passive muscle stiffness of short hamstrings. Arch Phys Med Rehabil 1996;77:658–92.

37. Hurtig DE, Henderson JM. Increasing hamstring flexibility decreases lower extremity overuse injuries in military basic trainees. Am J Sports Med 1999;27:173–6.

38. Thacker SB, Gilchrist J, Stroup DF, et al. The impact of stretching on sports injury risk: a systematic review of the literatures. Med Sci Sports Exerc 2004;36:371–8.

39. Herbert RD, Gabriel M. Effects of stretching before and after exercising on muscle soreness and risk of injury: systematic review. Br Med J 2002;325:468.

40. Shier I. Stretching before exercise does not reduce the risk of local muscle injury: a critical review of the clinical and basic science literature. Clin J Sport Med 1999;9:221–7.

41. Shrier I. Does stretching improve performance? A systematic and critical review of the literature. Clin J Sport Med 2004;14:267–73.

42. Murphy DR. A critical look at static stretching: are we doing our patient harm. Chiropractic Sports Med 1991;5:67–70.

43. Wilbur RL, Moffatt RJ, Scott BE, et al. Influence of water run training on the maintenance of aerobic performance. Med Sci Sports Exerc 1996;28(8):1056–62.

44. Ballas MT, Tytko J, Cookson D. Common overuse running injuries: diagnosis and management. Am Fam Physician 1997;55(7):2473–80.

45. Fredericson M, Moore W, Guillet M, et al. High hamstring tendonopathy in runners: meeting the challenges of diagnosis, treatment and rehabilitation. Phys Sportsmed 2005;33(5):32–43.

46. Borg G. Borg's Perceived Exertion and Pain Scales. Champaign (IL): Human Kinetics 1998.

47. Koplan JP, Powell KE, Sikes RK, et al. An epidemiologic study of the benefits and risks of running. JAMA 1982;248(23):3118–21.

48. Jacobs SJ, Berson BL. Injuries to runners: a study of entrants to a 10,000 meter race. Am J Sports Med 1986;14(2):151–5.

49. Fields KB, Sykes JC, Walker KM, et al. Prevention of running injuries. Curr Sports Med Rep 2010;9(3):176–82.

50. Messier SP, Legault C, Schoenlank CR, et al. Risk factors and mechanisms of knee injury in runners. Med Sci Sports Exerc 2008;40(11):1873–9.

51. Messier SP, Edwards DG, Martin DF, et al. Etiology of iliotibial band friction syndrome in distance runners. Med Sci Sports Exerc 1995;27(7):951–60.

52. Lee TG, Ahmad TS. Intralesional autologous blood injection compared to corticosteroid injection for treatment of chronic plantar fasciitis: a prospective, randomized, controlled trial. Foot Ankle Int 2007;28:984–90.

53. Porter MD, Shadbolt B. Intralesional corticosteroid injection versus extracorporeal shock wave therapy for plantar fasciopathy. Clin J Sport Med 2005;15:119–24.

54. Torkki M, Malmivaara A, Seitsalo S, et al. Surgery vs orthosis vs watchful waiting for hallux valgus: a randomized controlled trial. JAMA 2001;285(19):2474–80.

55. Torkki M, Malmivaara A, Seitsalo S, et al. Hallux valgus: immediate operation versus 1 year of waiting with or without orthoses: a randomized controlled trial of 209 patients. Acta Orthop Scand 2003;74(2):209–15.

56. Eiff MP, Smith AT, Smith GE. Early mobilization versus immobilization in the treatment of lateral ankle sprains. Am J Sports Med 1994;22(1):83–8.

57. Dettori JR, Basmania CJ. Early ankle mobilization, Part II: a one-year follow-up of acute, lateral ankle sprains (a randomized clinical trial). Mil Med 1994;159(1):20–4.

58. Karlsson J, Lundin O, Lind K, et al. Early mobilization versus immobilization after ankle ligament stabilization. Scand J Med Sci Sports 1999;9(5):299–303.

59. Wolfe MW, Uhl TL, Mattacola CG, et al. Management of ankle sprains. Am Fam Physician 2001;63(1):93–104 [erratum in: Am Fam Physician 2001;64(3):386].

60. Hartsell HD, Spaulding SJ. Eccentric/concentric ratios at selected velocities for the invertor and evertor muscles of the chronically unstable ankle. Br J Sports Med 1999;33(4):255–8.

61. Primack S. Ultrasound-guided foot/ankle procedures. Presented at AAPMR Diagnostic and Interventional Musculoskeletal Ultrasound of the Lower Extremity course. Las Vegas (NV), February, 2011.
62. Doucette SA, Goble EM. The effect of exercise on patellar tracking in lateral patellar compression syndrome. Am J Sports Med 1992;20:434–40.
63. Tyler TF, et al. The role of hip muscle function in the treatment of patellofemoral pain syndrome. Am J Sports Med 2006;34(4):630–6.
64. Nyland J, Lachman N, Kocabey Y, et al. Anatomy, function, and rehabilitation of the popliteus musculotendinous complex. J Orthop Sports Phys Ther 2005;35(3):165–79.
65. Fredericson M, White JJ, MacMahon JM, et al. Quantitative analysis of the relative effectiveness of 3 iliotibial band stretches. Arch Phys Med Rehabil 2002;83:589–92.
66. Fredericson M, Weir A. Practical management of iliotibial band friction syndrome in runners. Clin J Sport Med 2006;16(3):261–8.
67. Koulouris G, Connell D. Evaluation of the hamstring muscle complex following acute injury. Skeletal Radiol 2003;32:582–9.
68. Askling CM, Tengvar M, Saartok T, et al. Acute first-time hamstring strains during high-speed running: a longitudinal study including clinical and magnetic resonance imaging findings. Am J Sports Med 2007;35:197–206.
69. Brockett CL, Morgan DL, Proske U. Human hamstring muscles adapt to eccentric exercise by changing optimum length. Med Sci Sports Exerc 2001;33:783–90.
70. Orchard J, Best TM, Verrall GM. Return to play following muscle strains. Clin J Sport Med 2005;15:436–41.
71. Sherry MA, Best TM. A comparison of 2 rehabilitation programs in the treatment of acute hamstring strains. J Orthop Sports Phys Ther 2004;34:116–25.
72. Bennell K, Tully E, Harvey N. Does the toe-touch test predict hamstring injury in Australian Rules footballers? Aust J Physiother 1999;45:103–9.
73. Malliaropoulos N, Papalexandris S, Papalada A, et al. The role of stretching in rehabilitation of hamstring injuries: 80 athletes follow-up. Med Sci Sports Exerc 2004;36:756–9.
74. Mason DL, Dickens V, Vail A. Rehabilitation for hamstring injuries. Cochrane Database Syst Rev 2007;1:CD004575.
75. Levine WN, Bergfeld JA, Tessendorf W, et al. Intramuscular corticosteroid injection for hamstring injuries. A 13-year experience in the National Football League. Am J Sports Med 2000;28(3):297–300.
76. Nelson RT. A Comparison of the immediate effects of eccentric training vs static stretch on hamstring flexibility in high school and college athletes. N Am J Sports Phys Ther 2006;1(2):56–61.
77. Vitanzo PC Jr, McShane JM. Osteitis pubis: solving a perplexing problem. Phys Sportsmed 2001;29(7):33–48.
78. Lynch SA, Renström PA. Groin injuries in sport: treatment strategies. Sports Med 1999;28(2):137–44.
79. Holt MA, Keene JS, Graf BK, et al. Treatment of osteitis pubis in athletes. Results of corticosteroid injections. Am J Sports Med 1995;23(5):601–6.
80. Topol GA, Reeves KD, Hassanein KM. Efficacy of dextrose prolotherapy in elite male kicking-sport athletes with chronic groin pain. Arch Phys Med Rehabil 2005;86(4):697–702.
81. Lacroix VJ. A complete approach to groin pain. Phys Sportsmed 2000;28(1):66–86.
82. Philippon MJ, Decker MJ, Giphart JE, et al. Rehabilitation exercise progression for the gluteus medius muscle with consideration for iliopsoas tendinitis: an in vivo electromyography study. Am J Sports Med 2011;39(8):1777–85.

83. Moen MH, Tol JL, Weir A, et al. Medial tibial stress syndrome: a critical review. Sports Med 2009;39(7):523–46.
84. Touliopolous S, Hershman EB. Lower leg pain. Diagnosis and treatment of compartment syndromes and other pain syndromes of the leg. Sports Med 1999;27(3):193–204.
85. Moen MH, Bongers T, Bakker EW, et al. Risk factors and prognostic indicators for medial tibial stress syndrome. Scand J Med Sci Sports 2010. [Epub ahead of print].
86. Raissi GR, Cherati AD, Mansoori KD, et al. The relationship between lower extremity alignment and Medial Tibial Stress Syndrome among non-professional athletes. Sports Med Arthrosc Rehabil Ther Technol 2009;1(1):11.

Index

Note: Page numbers of article titles are in **boldface** type.

A

Achilles enthesopathy, 363–364
Achilles tendinopathy, 363–364
Achilles tendon, complete tear of, 226–227, 228
  hypoxic tendinosis of, 222, 225
  normal-sized, 220–221, 224
  overuse injuries of, in runners, 220–227
  tendinosis of, 221–222, 225
Ankle, and foot, in running, 192–193
Ankle inversion and eversion studies, in medial tibial stress syndrome, 277
Ankle joint, ranges of motion in running, 193
Ankle sprains, in runners, treatment of, 362–363
Anti-inflammatories, in tendinopathy, 330–332
Aprotinin, in tendinopathy, 339
Arm swing, during running gait cycle, 196, 197
Autologous whole blood, in tendinopathy, 336–337
Avulsion hamstring stress, 229, 233

B

Balance testing, and core stability testing, of injured runners, 211–213
    shoewear and, 212–213
Balance training, in running injuries, 358–359
Barefoot running, 212–213
  disadvantages of, 213
Biceps femoris, injury to, 228
Biophosphates, in bone diseases, 302–303
Bone, stress injury to, 217–219
Bone mineral density, and female athlete triad, 250–251
  low, stress fractures in, 292
Bone stimulators, in running injuries, 354
Bracing, in running injuries, 355

C

Calf injuries, rehabilitation following, 367–368
Cavus foot, 209–210
Compartment syndrome, exertional, 230–235
    chronic, **307–319**
      complications of, 316
      diagnostic testing in, 310–312
      evaluation in, 309–310

Clin Sports Med 31 (2012) 373–379
doi:10.1016/S0278-5919(12)00011-7
0278-5919/12/$ – see front matter © 2012 Elsevier Inc. All rights reserved.

Printed and bound by CPI Group (UK) Ltd, Croydon, CR0 4YY

03/10/2024

01040459-0019